Posthuman

Consciousness and Pathic Engagement

Posthuman

Consciousness and Pathic Engagement

Edited by

Mauro Maldonato and Paolo Augusto Masullo

sussex

2 4 6 8 10 9 7 5 3 1

First published in 2017 in Great Britain by
SUSSEX ACADEMIC PRESS
PO Box 139
Eastbourne BN24 9BP

Distributed in North America by
SUSSEX ACADEMIC PRESS
Independent Publishers Group
814 N Franklin St, Chicago, IL 60610, USA

British Library Cataloguing in Publication Data
A CIP catalogue record for this book is available from the British Library.

Library of Congress Cataloging-in-Publication Data
Names: Maldonato, Mauro, editor.
Title: Posthuman : consciousness and pathic engagement / edited by Mauro
    Maldonato and Paolo Augusto Masullo.
Description: Portland, Oregon : Sussex Academic Press, 2017. | Includes
    bibliographical references and index.
Identifiers: LCCN 2017014800 | ISBN 9781845197131 (pbk : alk. paper)
Subjects: LCSH: Humanism—History—21st century. | Humanism—
    Forecasting. | Philosophical anthropology.
Classification: LCC B821 .P59 2017 | DDC 144—dc23
LC record available at https://lccn.loc.gov/2017014800

Typeset & designed by Sussex Academic Press, Brighton & Eastbourne.

Contents

Acknowledgments

The Editors gratefully acknowledge the assistance of the Department of Human Sciences (DISU), University of Basilicata, Dr Luisa Caiazzo, and Dr Michelle Mennuni.

Our thanks to Roy Boardman, the translator, for his excellent work.

Introduction

MAURO MALDONATO AND PAOLO AUGUSTO MASULLO

Consciousness is the last and latest development of the organic and
hence also what is most unfinished and unstrong [...]
One thinks that it constitutes the kernel of man; what is abiding,
eternal, ultimate and most original in him [...]
(F. Nietzsche, *FW*, af. 11, 1882)

For a few decades, the spectre of a posthuman and postbiological future
has haunted cultural, philosophical and scientific studies of the contemporary world. The concerns (and, in other respects, enthusiasms)
springing from the idea that current technologies might take us beyond
mere biological improvements are being supported and fuelled by the
rapidly increasing capability of bio-engineering and information technologies. The hybridization of humans and machines – which has
divided scholarship into technophobes and technophiles and is certainly
not a recent phenomenon – calls for innovative reflections. Hence, the
question about man is no longer "what is man?", but rather "what is
man becoming?". A radically different issue.

In traditional theoretical research, manifesto ideas have made their
appearance, which are triggering several questions: is the crisis of the
human (seen as the organic being dominated more and more by the
inorganic) perhaps leading to new forms of disembodied subjectivities,
"machinic non-mechanic" in nature? Are we perhaps close to creating
artificial intelligences with cognitive abilities and a consciousness similar to our own? Even more than that: if machines get to be
increasingly more like men, will men in turn come to be more like
machines? It seems evident that in the well-established criticism of the
traditional anthropological perspective, a new evolutionary space is
opening up, where *bios* opposes *techne* in different ways. As fixist
ideas about the essence of man have waned, new features of the human
are emerging. The anthropological model itself, by which the human is
framed, seems to be worth considering, in both unitary and dynamic
terms, from a complex perspective, by virtue of the multiplicity of sci-

ences that man *shapes* and *is shaped* by. Contemporary man's staggering bio-techno-poietic activity seems, by inexorable virtualisation, self-disclosure and continual crossing over the boundaries of the real, to be driving him towards developments that, given his organic nature, are unpredictable.

As developments in the direction of biotechnological hybridization rapidly occur, the eradication of the human is becoming more and more feasible in terms of operational cognition and less and less so in affective-emotional terms. The importance of such a radical metamorphosis jeopardises not so much the presumptuous notion of "classical-modern" rationality, as the undeniable heritage of reason as being radically embedded in "sensitive" modes of feeling, that is "affective logics" whereby affections are ruled and governed. "Every passion contains its own quantum of reason", Nietzsche suggested, and "reason itself is a state of relations between different passions" which turns us into acting *individuals*, subjects of decisions, desiring and aware "erotic subjects", exactly by virtue of those "modes of feeling". Should we then wonder to what extent "technological mediation" will be able to be *trans-formative*, given that it is at the same time *preservative*, and hence able to make man capable of going *beyond* himself by preserving him? In fact, every act of *overcoming* cannot but be preservation, because should man not preserve himself in the act of overcoming, he would end up being *other-than-man*, an outcome resulting in a "fracture".

It is worth adding that over the long and winding path of evolution, the human brain has evolved into a complex architecture regulating and controlling the human body. The progressive acquisition of functions and competencies such as manual skills and verbal language – which go well beyond mere coordination of movement and feeding, attacking or escaping strategies – has enhanced an increasingly strong interaction with brain function, which has led to the mastering of communicative activities, instrumental techniques and abstract-symbolic thinking. The intertwining of these functions with more archaic ones, such as emotions, has been widely represented in all survival essential strategies, especially in (self)awareness. Hence, since the very beginning, brain functions and the human body have been all one and the same, only a bold abstraction might therefore allow us to distinguish between rational intelligence and emotive and bodily intelligence, which are both an outcome of *natural logics* whose rules have provided an evolutionary advantage. This means that human intelligence is an expression of co-evolutive demands and activities, in that any environmental changes require species adaptation and, in turn, any species variations affect environmental changes.

Decision making, especially at times of uncertainty and doubt, is what our brain does most of the time, according to rules that are different from those of formal logic inference models (extremely expensive and not always appropriate for decision-making problems). The great adaptive value of our emotional repertoire has played a key role so far whenever we are in danger or when hesitating or reflecting on what to do might turn out to be fatal. On the other hand, if, in order to meet the challenges posed by a hostile, unknown and unpredictable environment, our ancestors had relied on the subtle and sophisticated geometries of reason, we would probably not be here, judging from our development so far. Although the pressures faced by human beings at the dawn of civilization are no longer impelling at present, our "emotional mind" continues to be our sixth sense for identifying danger.

The history of artificial intelligence is completely different, quite the opposite in many respects. Since the very beginning, its objective has been to reproduce human rationality artificially, at the expense of such emotions as aggression, love, wonder, hate and so on. By neglecting body and environment on the one hand, and foregrounding reason on the other hand, the artificial intelligence project has laid the foundations for creating a mind without a body, an intelligence without interaction with the world seen as a pointless source of "noise". No concerns about survival issues or reproductive success. No need for emotional adaptation. No laborious reflections on ourselves or the other. An aseptic, semantically void environment. The only link between machines and the real world being a programme: an umbilical cord impenetrable to the world's unpredictable impact. This is one of the reasons why artificial intelligence can easily deal with and solve formal logical and mathematical problems, but not those problems that require creativity, improvisation, building and interpreting narratives, linguistic interpretations and the like.

Having said that, by its use of complex models, artificial intelligence has allowed us to reflect upon cognition without awareness, emotions and affectivity; to gather, by analogy, features apparently obvious though elusive; to understand, by contrast, the importance of the body and consciousness. On this basis, versatile and flexible artefacts are being built (humanoids, androids, robots, whatever we name them), characterised by intelligence placed in artificial bodies that are provided with sensory devices.

But are we talking about intelligent or conscious machines? Before answering this question, we need to make some preliminary considerations. Creating artificial entities that, like man, are able to think and experience feelings, emotions and events has, from being a science-fiction or cinematographic dream, has turned into a primary research goal. Just a few years ago, the general interest lay exclusively in reproducing those cognitive activities that characterise some species as being intelligent, above all the human species. From an engineering point of view, for a long time consciousness related qualitative and subjective issues have been neglected which, by virtue of their nature, could not be explained in objective and scientific terms. However, in recent years new directions are being explored. After a first wave of enthusiasm, it seemed evident that traditional artificial intelligence was not capable of reproducing a subject with all his features, therefore researchers came to the conclusion that it was essential first to understand the biological mechanisms underlying consciousness.

For a very long time, the question of consciousness has attracted and exasperated the minds of whoever may have tried to untangle its secrets, thus giving rise to alternate feelings, ranging from passionate enthusiasm to seductive disorientation and gloomy scepticism. However, what has turned consciousness into the mystery of mysteries? And why, for such a long time, have so many scholars found it hard to accept that at its core there is a neurobiological cortico-subcortical process, established by evolution, that has led to the distinction between the Self and the Other? And there are many reasons for this. For millennia, mysticism and materialism, metaphysics and ontology have played a crucial role. Fortunately, times are changing. As a result, neuroscientists increasingly agree on the possibility of facing the consciousness problem experimentally. Hence, the coming years will be decisive for the development of a new discipline whereby the methodological tools necessary for an understanding of the nature of consciousness can eventually be defined. At present, current science still ignores the extent to which a physical system can generate conscious experiences. In fact, it is not even able to explain the nature of this phenomenon, what it is that produces consciousness; whether consciousness is limited or can be expanded. The point is that being conscious is different from being alive, because whereas being alive means being made up of molecules based on DNA replication, being conscious means experiencing the world. It seems evident that we need deeper insights into these issues; furthermore, the difficulties we face may depend not so much on the issue itself, but on the hypotheses that are accepted about the very nature of reality. This is not the place to discuss this, yet it seems worth pointing out that if we are willing to reconsider our categories and notions, we have also to analyse the meaning of the term 'consciousness', a term that designates both the highest expressions of man's mind and his normal waking activity. Is such a term still appropriate to refer to phenomena that are so different from each other?

At present, having failed to reproduce subjects resembling human beings, researchers seem to be attempting to reproduce the brain's basic mechanisms in order to duplicate the conscious subject. Needless to say, the rise of artificial intelligence machines is closely linked to the possibility of overcoming the critical threshold of complexity. And this is not only related to whether or not the huge endeavours underlying thousands of years of history can be replicated, but also to whether there is any possibility of addressing the longstanding bioethic debate about the consequences of such an enterprise. Is it possible to circumvent these obstacles? Are there any viable alternatives to revolutionising our fundamental cultural categories, which, by means of a new method, would enable us to integrate both subjective and objective dimensions, so that the former do not necessarily have to be reduced to the latter? Until now, attempts have been made to address the consciousness issue by reliance on Galilean categories, which have proved very successful at explaining physical phenomena, but inadequate to explain mental ones. When a human being experiences the world (i.e., perceives colours and tastes or feels pain or pleasure), he/she is experiencing qualitative features of reality that Galilean science is not able to explain. Perhaps building something whose founding principles are unknown might be a way to shed light on them.

A deeper understanding of our consciousness would allow us not only to get to the bottom of our own relationship with it, but also to see how fast the future is approaching. A fresh view of this sphere would have a substantial effect on us. Ancient doubts on human identities and freedoms would be revived and so no longer be at risk of being filed away as though they were the remains of a declining civilization, doomed to be replaced by a future characterised by the presence of human-looking organisms, who might look at us as we look in such amazement at fossils from the African savannah. As a point in fact, it is widely believed that the encounter between man and highly-powered computers will, sooner or later, generate organisms capable of going well beyond the simulation of cerebral functions: hybrids who will learn from their inner states, interpret data from reality, define their own objectives, talk with us humans; above all they will make decisions based on their own 'system of values'. In a not too distant future, these organisms might even achieve broader and broader spheres of autonomy, self-preserving needs, hierarchies of values, possibly an ethics based on "freedom". Undoubtedly, it will be very difficult to continue to think of experience as information processing (however sophisticated it may be), or to call emotions pain and pleasure. But can we really exclude the possibility that one day these entities might have a spirit of enterprise, of initiative, and be able to exercise discernment?

We should not, however, be alarmed by our present inability to answer these questions. Quite the opposite, we should feel encouraged to explore these issues from unusual perspectives. Furthermore, building artefacts might help us to ask the right questions in order to understand principles that we have not yet grasped. It would help us to expand the boundaries of a map of reality that is at present still beyond our reach and allow us to draw new ones. Would such an approach involve taking risks or making mistakes? Very likely. So what? Are all our attempts at knowledge not likely to be at risk or doomed to failure? Are our truths anything other than provisional and conjectural? Conjectures and failures are not accidental to knowledge: even though they are in the background, they do nonetheless play an essential role. If we do care about finding out the regularity of phenomena, then we should also care about all that is indemonstrable and inaccessible in relation to them. So, we will be able to face both our fears and our ambitions, keeping aside any rhetoric of intransigence, without idolizing any ideology, be it living tissue physics, or conscious silicon. Because such an attitude would undermine not only the rigour of our research but also the boldness of our questions.

These reflections have provided the starting point for the present book, which brings together contributions of scholars from different countries and professional backgrounds/disciplinary fields. The thread that links the scientific enquiries and perspectives represented is the shared need for a critical view of the *homo bio-technologicus* ideology. In order to preserve his human dimension, this "new man", increasingly powerful owing to his singularity, and at the same time manifold as a result of his growing hybridizing capability, "has to" *trespass-himself* through technology, but he "cannot" transform himself, in the sense of denying himself; he has rather, less ambitiously, to "betray" himself in the sense of *translate* himself in order to become "more than human": not an anthropocentric and self-referential being, but in this sense, a pluricentric ethero-referential being. A "new man" also means "new *ethos*", hence a man capable, also by virtue of his own heightened *pathe*, of will, power, duty and abilities, a man able to morally come-to-terms with any *alterity* by becoming "ultra-human", that is "more-than-human", thus relying on a new hermeneutics of his modes of feeling. In conclusion, in spite of his new performative abilities, *homo biotechnologicus* cannot give up building a new landscape of affections. This is why the "pathosophie of the posthuman" is needed.

1

Robots as Post-humans: Some Issues about Artificial Life

SANTO F. DI NUOVO AND DANIELA CONTI

The chapter deals with the possibility of recognizing the quality of 'awareness' in post-human forms, as robotics and artificial life.

Today the powerful means of neuroscience, combined with those of artificial intelligence and robotics, allow us to create simulations of life that build an "intelligent post-human".

In robotics, brain and body are connected in a unity: while information technologies are "disembodied" (Hayles 1999), robotics permits to simulate a mind resident inside a body, including the possibility of *mind uploading*; that is, reproducing artificial models faithful to the original that behave like as the human embodied mind (Sandberg/Boström 2008).

How these goals of post-human life can be reached at best?

What is – if available – the 'awareness' of these embodied artificial minds?

1. Genetic Algorithms for an 'Intelligent' Adaptation

Algorithms called "genetic" are related to the natural evolution and therefore to the Darwinian principles of selection, reproduction and mutation. The simulation starts with the search for solutions to the specific problem considered, evaluates for each of these solutions the fitness or ability to carry out adjustments, recombines them iteratively introducing elements of disorder with the aim of creating new solutions, reaching the best one possible in relation to the environmental conditions.

It is well known that, using genetic algorithms, models of the selective reproduction of individuals can be generated, identifying groups more efficient in adapting, implementing the 'crossover' or genetic recombination, including random mutations; ultimately it is possible to simulate life in its phylogenetic evolution. These strategies of artificial reproduction of life can realize an optimal genetic development, generating populations of organisms that learn and reproduce in a specific environment, selecting themselves based on the ability to adapt to it.

No form of awareness is required for this genetic development, which can be defined as 'intelligent' to the extent that it is useful to realize advanced forms of adaptation.

2. Reproducing Ontogenesis: Epigenetic Changes in Lifespan

What happens when we try to reproduce activities that characterize the typically human development? Trying to artificially replicate aspects of life that affect sensory perception, sensory-motor coordination, recognition of images and words, identification of appropriate emotions in a context, means to mimic ontogenetic adaptability, that is, the individuals in relation to their environment (Cangelosi/Schlesinger 2015).

The experiences and learned competencies of the organism are essential for its adaptive development. They have to be simulated by appropriate techniques: the Artificial Neural Networks have proven to be capable of reproducing operation of the psychobiologic systems on which learning is based.

When we try to reproduce real life – unlike the first simplified simulations – we have to take into account the interaction between organisms sharing the same environment; thus including the emotional and bodily aspects that psychology has shown to be constitutive of the social relations. In a neuro-constructivist approach, genes, neural networks, and social behavior actively interact for producing ontogenetic changes (Dekker/Karmiloff-Smith 2011).

Within the ontogenesis also epigenetic components are included, an important and timely object of study in the life sciences. Through *epigenetics* (studying the gene as it evolves in the environment, and not as a fixed entity), the brain and the embodied mind can be understood not only as the result by default of a fixed genetic program; the functionality of the genes can change, based on external stimuli. An enriching environment (i.e., stimuli for sensation, perception, motivation, emotion) can determine "epi-mutations": changes in genetic functioning, while the basic structure remains unchanged (Changeux 1983, Wong/Craig 2011, Spector 2012).

There is experimental evidence on the effects of enriched environments in determining the neuronal plasticity (i.e., changes in functioning and adaptation): while the genetic specification guides the initial processes of brain development and the formation of neural connections, the particular experience of the individual and the interactions with the environment, more or less rich in stimulation, lead to adjust the final stages of development. The organism can retrieve some impaired functions, not only in the early development but even at an advanced stage of lifespan (Huttenlocher 2002, Sale/Berardi/Maffei 2009, 2014).

3. Can Artificial Life Reproduce Human Life?

The *Artificial Life*, the last frontier of the Artificial Intelligence, involves the construction of organisms comparable to living beings, capable not only of replicating genetically at best, but also to survive, reproduce and independently develop complex social and cognitive functions (Di Nuovo/Cangelosi 2015). This approach necessarily involves the interaction between different sciences – biology, ethology, sociology, psychology, neuroscience, chemistry, computer science, engineering and materials science – extending beyond disciplinary boundaries toward a "General Theory of Life".

An artificial organism has to perform tasks comparable to those performed by living organisms, from insects to small animals to humans. To achieve this comparability, we need mechanisms based on realistic physics, sensors deliberately imperfect (as natural ones) and living in an environment full of 'noise', that is of intervening variables that cannot be eliminated, just those typical of the real life: never similar to a laboratory, where complexity can be reduced and noise eliminated.

Building an automatic apparatus showing an adaptive behavior is a goal of engineering: it was done in 2001, inspired by the ideas of Tolman about the artificial *oniscus*, that the author in 1939 had not been able to realize for lack of technological means (Endo/Arkin 2001, Miglino/Gigliotta/Cardaci/Ponticorvo 2007). Beyond the technological aims of engineering, the purpose of achieving psychological and social goals broadens the range of possible applications of artificial life.

In simulating life attitudes we have to implement the interpersonal and group relationships, the theories of the mind and the phenomena of empathy or prejudice, the values of cooperation or competition, the processes used for self-regulation, links and conflicts, considering also the external conditions, as suggested by the "social neuroscience" (Harmon-Jones/Winkielman 2007).

In this perspective the theory of "extended mind" (Menary 2010) includes the environment in which the mind finds continuous and vital exchanges. The expanding of the mind in the world should be taken into account when we try to reproduce the living phenomena in artificial systems: from the computerized simulations of relations, to the construction of physical systems that add to the artificial mind the dimension of the body, such as robots and automatons. The developmental models, studying the variations of systems that selectively reproduce themselves, integrating new variations, may account reliably – albeit simulated – the complexity of biological but also cultural evolution. Starting from simple simulations of single-celled organisms it is possible to get complex models and artificial organisms, related to social and organizational interactions characterizing the interpersonal mind and the social life.

These complex models, beyond the aim of implementing scientific knowledge, can be used to build assistive technologies for supporting – in an 'intelligent' way – the humans in the post-human era.

4. Can Artificial Intelligence Helps Humans? Assistive Robotics in Social Settings

The definition "Socially Assistive Robotics" (SAR) covers an interdisciplinary field that combines engineering, medicine and psychology, and has a wide range of present and possible applications. Its essential characteristic is the social interaction as a means to help the persons with special needs, not as a substitute for specialized and competent professionals, neither as a panacea for all the needs of mental health. The robot, as embodied mind dynamically acting in social contexts, could be a useful tool to support various clinical and assistive conditions.

- In the field of education and care of children, SAR was successfully applied to help health education of children with diabetes (Blanson Henkemans *et al.* 2013); to assist either teachers in telling pre-recorded stories to preschool children (Fridin 2014) or parents in home education (Han *et al.* 2005).
- In clinical settings, Beran, Ramirez-Serrano, Vanderkooi, and Kuhn (2013) has shown how human–robot interaction can be used as a medium for pediatric care, e.g. to use cognitive-behavioural, distraction, and coaching strategies to support children during various types of medical procedures such as tissue repair, intravenous starts, oral hygiene and dental treatments, etc.

- Elderly people with and without mental deterioration have a good acceptation of assistive social robotics, which therefore be widely used for caring with the supervision of human programmers (Broekens/Heerink/Rosendal 2009, Chen/Chan, 2011, Fasola/Matarić 2010, Klamer/Ben Allouch 2010). An European project – "Implementation and integration of advanced *Robot*ic systems and intelligent *E*nvironments in *r*eal scenarios for the *a*geing population", i.e., *Robot-Era* project – aims to assist elderly in the daily life, at home and in social contexts (Di Nuovo *et al.* 2014).
- Physical rehabilitation (e.g., after a stroke or sport trauma) can be enhanced by artificially reproducing the principles of posture and movement and using them in technological supports to rehabilitation (Fasola/Matarić 2012 and 2013, Matarić /Eriksson/ Feil-Seifer/Winstein 2007, Tăpuş/ Tăpuş /Matarić 2008).
- In intellectual disability (also at severe levels) some cognitive, motor and social skills can be improved with the help of artificial intelligence (Houwen/van der Putten/Vlaskamp 2014, Tăpuş/ Tăpuş/Matarić 2009).
- The use of robots as companions for educational games and support for professionals has been proven useful also in attention disorders, with and without hyperactivity (Fridin/Yaakobi 2011) and in Down syndrome (Lehmann *et al.* 2014).
- The robot as assistive tool in psychological therapies can help to develop new social behaviors in adults with mental pathologies and in children with developmental disorders such as autism (Diehl, Schmitt, Villano, & Crowell 2012, Feil-Seifer/Matarić 2009, Robins/Dautenhahn/Boekhorst/Billard 2005, Scassellati/ Henny Admoni/Matarić 2012).

The humanoid robot NAO, popular for its ease of use and adaptability to different contexts of therapy and rehabilitation, suitable for working with children with atypical development even in scholastic contexts, has proved very useful in the stimulation of imitative behavior in children with autism and moderate to severe intellectual disabilities (Shamsuddin *et al.* 2012a; Thill *et al.* 2013). In the Shamsuddin's *et al.* study (2012b), after a planned interaction between NAO and autistic children with impaired intelligence, four out of five children exhibited a decrease of autistic behavior, mainly regarding communication: the robot was able to attract the children's attention, keep each child engaged during interaction and hence give positive impact to the children's communication behavior. Along the same line of research, some preliminary results have been presented in a pilot study with three children with autism and intellectual disability (Conti *et al.* 2015). The pilot study focused on imitation skills, and the analysis of the results suggested that the assistive technology can be an effective tool to support established psychological therapies for autism.

5. The Autonomy of the Artificial and the Problem of 'Control'

The grounding basis, shared by all these technological applications of artificial life, is that artificial organisms initially selected and trained by external inputs, in their development can use also *internal* resources: i.e. knowledge, acquired schemes, even motivational drives as autonomous search for planned goals.

These inner resources become somehow independent from external stimuli and 'work inside' in a recursive way, with a kind of purposeful and teleological awareness of means-end relations, and with a capacity of self-controlling and self-adapting: this ability could be called *'conscience'* of the artificial. Obviously, the term should be intended with all the limits implied by its philosophical meaning, and recognizing the possibility that humans continue to plan and verify the action of the artificial organism when using it for assistive goals.

The capacity of self-control and self-regulation of an artificial system has been defined in Wiener's theory of cybernetics as a continuous minimizing of the error, reducing the gap between the present state of the system and the desired goal. The ability to achieve the same objective in self-monitoring toward a higher-level goal (*consciousness*?) can be added.

The question is whether this 'leap' of order of the final goal can really come from *within* the system or must still be pre-ordered *from the outside* (by genetics and/or by relevant, or binding, external events). Could have the intelligent machine an internal means-end planning system capable of changing in time, starting from procedures included a priori in the system itself, but not more depending on an outer control? May the system capacity to change its strategies also in an original way – having been trained for this aim, and to do this independently – extend to change the aims to which strategies are initially directed? Ultimately, the question is whether an artificial system, as well as learning how to work better than those who created it (which could be well accepted by humans), can independently develop a *heterogenesis of purposes*, that emerge from a chain of activities having initially different aims.

Therefore, a big problem arises: should these intelligent lives always have a human 'controller', who monitors the processes, as it already happens (although without cybernetic support) for educators, therapists, rehabilitators, financial analysts, meteorologists? Or can they, in turn, be entrusted to artificial systems acting as 'supervising controllers', which, taking advantage of increasingly powerful data processing capabilities of intelligent supercomputers, are able to monitor the evolution of the 'controlled' organism toward the predetermined objective?

This second possibility – i.e., the monitoring entity itself is artificial – is currently the subject of ambitious scientific projects and of literary or movie fictions; if realized, relevant problems of economic feasibility, and ethical and political issues, should be posed:

- Who will be able to sponsor, fund and organize these 'controller' systems of artificial life and therefore to manage all their power?
- Who (or what) will "guard the guardians" if these artificial agents will be capable of self-regulation and adaptation with regard also to possible modifications of the ultimate goals (according to the previously discussed heterogenesis of purposes)?

However, these essential questions arise also in the case in which the controllers remain human, even if sophisticated cybernetic systems are used to assist them.

6. The Need of a Theory of Intelligence and of Life for Building Intelligent Artificial Life

We have seen that a comprehensive theory of intelligence – not only cognitive but also motivational, emotional and similar to the real human practical intelligence – is needed to build intelligent agents capable to be accepted by humans as companions and help in their everyday life.

We have seen also that the possible heterogenesis of purposes is the main risk the humans see in artificial beings: this possibility includes an autonomous awareness of *what* to do and *how* to do in the interaction with humans, often hard to accept by humans themselves.[1]

We have seen that artificial life, the last frontier of the artificial intelligence, could lead to an unknown future for humanity if capable of autonomous and uncontrolled 'conscience'.

To define what is similar to the human in the post-human, and what can be considered as a 'conscience', it is important to define the assumptions and the theoretical coordinates appropriate to the complexity of the problem.

In the re-construction of life in artificial organisms the application of *theory-grounded* and *data-driven* models are combined.

- The first models start by the conclusions of both basic and applicative research regarding mind, embodied cognition, social neuroscience, cognitive sciences, anthropology and sociology. They use increasingly sophisticated genetic algorithms whose efficiency is tested in simulations, then extending 'in the field' the ones that work. Theories remain the ground for all the possible applications, and lead them 'a priori'.
- Instead, models derived from the data implement artificial organisms that replicate experimental observations. In this case we have 'emerging' structures, which include increasingly complex variables, thanks to the great power of updated computers. The purpose of the 'emergent' approach, as well as "remake reality in the computer", as proposed by the Palmer's book (2001), is to create new realities, reproducing (or simulating) the mechanisms of adaptation, learning and development, underlying the life of a biological system. Specific skills or behaviors are not directly imitated or reproduced, as schematic 'photographs' of a part of reality, or as direct applications of a theory, but emerge as a result of adaptation processes put in place by the new reality built artificially. This emergence and autonomous learning from the experience lead organisms to develop driven by the data acquired by itself, not by a background theory of the developer.

Traditionally, artificial life realizes models that *simulate* psychophysical activities: e.g., phenomena such as the *unilateral spatial neglect* (Conti, Di Nuovo S., Cangelosi, Di Nuovo A. 2016) or physical and/or psychic diseases, the characteristics of which are well known from experimental research. The assistive use of the artificial derives from these theoretical advances, which the artificial itself contributes to implement.

A different way is to create artificial organisms that *live* and *evolve* in the real world, autonomously adapting to concrete and specific environments.

To build a driving simulator in different environmental contexts we can start from a theoretical analysis of the functions that are used to drive well, varying applications in the different conditions of the subject and of the environment, using algorithms that are then verified in real settings, maintaining in the simulator those who 'work' best in the given conditions.

If we have to support elderly with deficits in functions of spatial orientation to find pathways needed for everyday life, we can refer to a scientific model of perception, attention, imagination and motor memory, and implement each key aspects of the model in the real environment by means of programmed *tags* or other 'intelligent' devices.

Another way is to build an environment of artificial life with some useful landmarks to facilitate the path, programmed in a functional way, and implementing artificial organism capable of verifying empirically whether the system is efficient for the proposed aim, modifying if necessary some aspects to fit the individual subject's needs. This building is facilitated by the technologies widely available and accessible to non-experts: even kids can build robots with the ability to move, speak, and evolve, through a Lego© construction kit, called *MindStorm*.

7. Conclusions and Future Directions

For all simulations related to individual and social learning, some basic bonds – perhaps contrasting each other – remain.

The artificial will have ecological validity only if it is compliant with the conditions of the environment and the context in which it is implemented and used; otherwise it remains in a laboratory field, whose extension to daily life will remain problematic.

As a consequence of the need to fit the complexity of the real context, the artificial should acquire autonomous 'consciousness', by means of recurrent neural networks, which do not need continuous external inputs and are capable of regulating their own feedbacks. This autonomy, and lack of necessity of outer control, could be dangerous for the future of the human beings: it will be a fearful post-human.

As a recent, and somehow perturbing, advance assigning consciousness to virtual reality, we will cite the possibility to reproduce the individual mind and to preserve it artificially in time and space, as claimed by the 'trans-humanist' or *Humanity+* approach (Bostrom 2005). Trans-humanism aims at creating a fusion of biology, cognitive science, computer science and nanotechnology to simulate and upload the individual consciousness on a digital support, creating a huge virtual database of conscious minds resistant over time.

According to the trans-humanist Ray Kurzweil (2005), transferring the individual consciousness in the web is a way of ensuring the survival after the end of life. The last step towards immortality is the possibility to create an ageless copy of themselves, in a database which would constitute a new virtual humanity, without spatial and temporal boundaries, in a simulated world living beyond death. The "2045 Initiative" (www.2045.com) aims at replacing bodies and brains, predisposed to frailty and death, with holographic people. Thus it would somehow overcome the end of the individual human life, realizing the potential immortality which is the aspiration of humanity since the beginning of the world: a desire translated into all the religions as belief in an afterlife, in the possibility of 're-incarnation', that simulation may now realize.

Ethical and religious critical positions are imaginable. Indeed, this kind of "life beyond life" would be planned and ruled by intelligent agents reproducing the very essence of life: the conscious mind. They will reproduce also the dangers of what has been called "cybernetic totalitarianism". Bostrom (2014) himself, a founder of trans-humanism, has recently warned against the risks that virtual intelligences overwhelming human intelligence could induce humanity to depend on the machines and create potential existential disasters: precisely the danger that, as we have seen, humans instinctively feel come from too smart humanoids.

For building artificial life in both 'ecological' and non-fearful way, what are the *theories of life* from which we can start, for the implementation and the subsequent verification?

Ultimately, *what kind of life* (including the issues of 'control') we want to simulate, and *why*?

Neural networks simulate biological functions based on neural models substantially shared in neuroscientific theories, thanks to more and more technologically efficient diagnostic tools. If we intend to simulate vital, existential functions, the required theoretical models are often quite different, as evidenced by the social, educational, clinical theories, often divergent even in their internal models. When the theoretical models are complex, dynamic, and often chaotic – that is, not predictable for the simultaneous interaction of many variables and the intervention of random conditions, the artificial intelligence should follow a specific 'open-ended' logic. The nonlinearity of life requires models and implementation methods that can meet these conditions, therefore leading an autonomous searching for new patterns of knowledge and action to cope with the new condition not included in the early planning.

The construction of artificial life can proceed progressively and controlling *in itinere*, monitoring and changing the developments, as happens in the natural life. This allows reassuring about the problem of 'control': humans continue to control the post-human – obviously, with all the ethical and political problems existing in this matter since the origins of the technology.

In an epistemological and methodological perspective, the dynamic complexity of living systems does not allow for reducing to serial and partial analyses of them, despite refined methods and technologies used.

When the systems are very complex, the applicative actions based on the artificial should continuously monitor the changes produced over time, orienting the change towards the prefigured goals, facing the chance variations that would radically deviate from the goals.

At the same time the *life sciences* (biological, clinical, psychological, social) should theorize appropriate models of life in its various phases and temporal dynamics, so that the artificial simulations are able to reproduce it, stimulating and orienting applications from which in turn human life can get real benefits; or, at least, are able to verify the match of emerging structures with suitable and accepted models of life.

Reciprocally, we have to understand what 'awareness' humans have of the artificial reality – particularly when it – as in robots – assumes a human-like shape. This issue will be addressed in chapter 6.

Note

1   This issue will be treated in the next chapter, including examples from literature and movies.

Bibliography

Beran, T. N., Ramirez-Serrano, A., Vanderkooi, O. G., Kuhn, S. 2013: Humanoid Robotics in Health Care: An Exploration of Children's and Parents' Emotional Reactions. *Journal of Health Psychology. Vaccine* 31 (25), 2772–2777.

Blanson Henkemans, O. A., Bierman, B. P. B., Janssen, J., Neerincx, M. A., Looije, R., van der Bosch, H., van der Giessen, J. A. M. 2013: Using a Robot to Personalise Health Education for Children with Diabetes Type 1: A Pilot Study. *Patient Education and Counseling* 92 (2), 174-181.

Bostrom N. 2005: A History of Transhumanist Thought. *Journal of Evolution and Technology* 14 (1), 1–25.

Bostrom N. 2014: *Superintelligence: Paths, Dangers, Strategies.* Oxford: University Press.

Broekens, J., Heerink, M., Rosendal, H. 2009: Assistive Social Robots in Elderly Care: A Review. *Gerontechnology* 8 (2), 94–103.

Cangelosi, A., Schlesinger, M. 2015: *Developmental Robotics: From Babies to Robots.* Cambridge: MIT Press/Bradford Books.

Changeux, J. P. 1983 : *L'homme neuronal.* Paris: Fayard.

Chen, K., Chan, H. S. 2011: A Review of Technology Acceptance by Older Adults. *Gerontechnology* 10 (1), 1–12.

Conti, D., Di Nuovo, S., Cangelosi, A., & Di Nuovo, A. (2016): Lateral Specialization in Unilateral Special Neglect: A Cognitive Robotics Model. *Cognitive Processing*, 17(3), 321–328.

Conti, D., Di Nuovo, S., Trubia, G., Buono, S., Di Nuovo, A. 2015: Use of Robotics to Stimulate Imitation in Children with Autism Spectrum Disorder: A Pilot Study in a Clinical Setting. In *RO-MAN, 2015 IEEE*, 1–6.

Dekker, T. M., Karmiloff-Smith, A. 2011: The Dynamics of Ontogeny: A Neurocostructivist Perspective on Genes, Brains, Cognition and Behavior. *Progress in Brain Research* 189, 23–33.

Diehl, J. J., Schmitt, L. M., Villano, M., Crowell, C. R. 2012: The Clinical Use of Robots for Individuals with Autism Spectrum Disorders: A Critical Review. *Research in Autism Spectrum Disorders* 6 (1), 249–262.

Di Nuovo, A., Broz, F., Belpaeme, T., Cangelosi, A., Cavallo, F., Esposito, R., Dario, P. 2014: A Web Based Multi-Modal Interface for Elderly Users of the Robot-Era Multi-robot Services. In *IEEE International Conference on Systems, Man and Cybernetics*. IEEE Press, 2186–2191.

Di Nuovo, S. Cangelosi, A. (eds) 2015: *Vita naturale, vita artificiale. Tecniche di simulazione e applicazioni educative e cliniche*. Milano: FrancoAngeli.

Endo Y., Arkin R. C. 2001: Implementing Tolman's Schematic Sowbug: Behavior-based Robotics in the 1930s. *Paper presented at the IEEE International Conference on Robotics and Automation (ICRA)* 1, 477–484.

Fasola, J., Matarić, M. J. 2010: Robot Exercise Instructor: A Socially Assistive Robot System to Monitor and Encourage Physical Exercise for the Elderly. In *RO-MAN, 2010 IEEE*, 416–421.

Fasola, J., Matarić, M. J. 2012: Using Socially Assistive Human–Robot Interaction to Motivate Physical Exercise for Older Adults. *Proceedings of the IEEE* 100 (8), 2512–2526.

Fasola, J., Matarić, M. J. 2013: Socially Assistive Robot Exercise Coach for the Elderly. *Journal of Human–Robot Interaction* 2, 3–32.

Feil-Seifer, D., Matarić, M. J. 2009: Toward Socially Assistive Robotics for Augmenting Interventions for Children with Autism Spectrum Disorders. In *Springer Tracts in Advanced Robotics* 54, 201–210.

Fridin, M. 2014: Storytelling by a Kindergarten Social Assistive Robot: A Tool for Constructive Learning in Preschool Education. *Computers and Education* 70, 53–64.

Han, J. H. J., Jo, M. J. M., Park, S. P. S., Kim, S. K. S. 2005: The Educational Use of Home Robots for Children. *IEEE International Workshop on Robot and Human Interactive Communication*.

Fridin, M., Yaakobi, Y. 2011: Educational Robot for Children with ADHD/ADD, Architecture Design. *Proceedings of International Conference on Computational Vision and Robotics*, Bhubaneswa, India.

Harmon-Jones, E., Winkielman, P. (eds) 2007: *Social Neuroscience. Integrating Biological and Psychological Explanation of Social Behavior*. New York: Guilford Press.

Hayles, N. K. 1999: *How we Became Posthuman: Virtual Bodies in Cybernetics, Literature, and Informatics*. Chicago: University Press.

Houwen, S., van der Putten, A., Vlaskamp, C. 2014: A Systematic Review of the Effects of Motor Interventions to Improve Motor, Cognitive, and/or Social Functioning in People with Severe or Profound Intellectual Disabilities. *Research in Developmental Disabilities* 35 (9), 2093–2116.

Huttenlocher, P. R. 2002: *Neural Plasticity: The Effects of Environment on the Development of the Cerebral Cortex*. Cambridge: Harvard University Press.

Klamer, T., Ben Allouch, S. 2010: Acceptance and Use of a Social Robot by Elderly Users in a Domestic Environment. In *4th International Conference on Pervasive Computing Technologies for Healthcare (PervasiveHealth)*,1–8.

Kurzweil R. 2005: *The Singularity is Near: When Humans Transcend Biology*. New York: Viking.

Lehmann, H., Iacono, I., Dautenhahn, K., Marti, P., Robins, B. 2014: Robot Companions for Children with Down Syndrome: A Case Study. *Interaction Studies* 15 (1), 99–112.

Matarić, M. J., Eriksson, J., Feil-Seifer, D. J., Winstein, C. J. 2007: Socially Assistive Robotics for Post-stroke Rehabilitation. *Journal of Neuroengineering and Rehabilitation* 4(1): 5.

Menary, R. (ed.) 2010: *The Extended Mind*. Cambridge: MIT Press/Bradford.

Miglino, O., Gigliotta, O., Cardaci, M., Ponticorvo, M. 2007: Artificial Organisms as Tools for the Development of Psychological Theory: Tolman's Lesson. *Cognitive Processing* 8 (4), 261–277.

Palmer, F. R. 2001: *Mood and Modality*. Cambridge: Cambridge University Press.

Robins, B., Dautenhahn, K., Boekhorst, R. T., Billard, A. 2005: Robotic Assistants in Therapy and Education of Children with Autism: Can a Small Humanoid Robot Help Encourage Social Interaction Skills? *Universal Access in the Information Society* 4 (2), 105–120.

Sale A., Berardi N., Maffei L. 2009: Enrich the Environment to Empower the Brain. *Trends in Neuroscience* 32 (4), 233–239.

Sale A., Berardi N., Maffei L. 2014: Environment and Brain Plasticity: Towards an Endogenous Pharmacotherapy. *Physiological Reviews* 94, 189–234.

Sandberg, A., Boström, N. 2008: *Whole Brain Emulation: A Roadmap*. Oxford: Future of Humanity Institute, Oxford University.

Scassellati, B., Admoni, H., Matarić, M. 2012: Robots for Use in Autism Research. *Annual Review of Biomedical Engineering* 14, 275–294.

Shamsuddin, S., Yussof, H., Ismail, L. I., Mohamed, S., Hanapiah, F. A., Zahari, N. I. 2012a: Initial Response in HRI – a Case Study on Evaluation of Child with Autism Spectrum Disorders Interacting with a Humanoid Robot NAO. *Procedia Engineering* 41, 1448–1455.

Shamsuddin, S., Yussof, H., Ismail, L. I., Mohamed, S., Hanapiah, F. A., Zahari, N. I. 2012b: Humanoid Robot NAO Interacting with Autistic Children of Moderately Impaired Intelligence to Augment Communication Skills. *Procedia Engineering* 41, 1533–1538.

Spector, T. 2012: *Identically Different: Why You Can Change Your Genes*. London: Weidenfeld & Nicolson.

Tăpuş, A., Tăpuş, C., Matarić, M. J. 2008: User-robot Personality Matching and Assistive Robot Behavior Adaptation for Post-stroke Rehabilitation Therapy. *Intelligent Service Robotics* 1 (2), 169–183.

Tapus, A., Tapus, C., Matarić, M. J. 2009: The Role of Physical Embodiment of a Therapist Robot for Individuals with Cognitive Impairments. In *Proceedings – IEEE International Workshop on Robot and Human Interactive Communication*, 103–107.

Thill, S., Pop, C., Belpaeme, T., Ziemke, T., Vanderborght, B. 2013: Robot-assisted Therapy for Autism Spectrum Disorders with (Partially) Autonomous Control: Challenges and Outlook. *Paladyn* 3 (4), 209–217.

Wong, N. C. Craig, J. M. 2011: *Epigenetics: A Reference Manual*. Norfolk: Caister.

2

Transsexualism as an Icon of Posthumanism: A Sartrean Critical Reconsideration

ROBERTO VITELLI

1. Introduction: Investigating Posthumanist Subjectivities

Recent developments in biotechnology and computer-based techniques have led to the possibility of enhancing, reproducing, reconstructing, substituting in the future, and more generally rethinking the human being as a new entity, no longer exclusively founded on 'carbon-based processes', but (also) on 'silicon-based ones': an entity combining non-organic matter with organic qualities, or exclusively bound up in cybernetic circuits or in now unthinkable possible different substrates or forms of life.[1] So Posthumanism and Transhumanism have emerged rapidly as new fields within the humanities and the social sciences.[2] The relationship between the two terms is quite controversial, as they are often wrongly used as synonyms. In fact, if, on the one hand, both spring from a reflection on the actual and/or futuristic impact of technology on life, on the other, they differ in many important ways. In a very general sense, transhumanists share some core humanist values and aspirations, like rationality, autonomy, compassion and aesthetic appreciation of human beings (Bostrom 2008), but they maintain that the traditional methods and ideas employed by humanists are limited in their scope by the material constraints of human biology and those of nature in a more general sense (Sorgner 2013, Habermas 2005). They state that actual and prospective developments of NBCI technologies (Nanotechnology, Biotechnology, Information Technology, and Cognitive Science) as well as biomedical technologies allow, and will increasingly allow in the future, an amplification and enhancement of human capacities and possibilities. In particular, they say, the extraordinary acceleration of technological advancement has today offered humans, and will offer them more and more in future, unprecedented control over their own nature and morphology. On the other hand, Posthumanism should more correctly be divided into two main conceptual categories: Critical Posthumanism and Speculative Posthumanism. Although both criticize human-centered (anthropocentric) ways of understanding life and reality, the latter opposes human-centric thinking about the long-term implications of modern technology, believing that in the future techno-logically-engendered nonhumans, as hypothetical wide "descendents" of current humans (Roden 2015), will probably experience and under-stand the world in ways that are today unpredictable as a consequence of some technological modification. Critical Posthumanism, on the contrary, is a broadly based attack on the supposed anthropocentrism of modern philosophy and intellectual life (Roden 2015): it "seeks to investigate the possible crisis and end of a certain conception of the human, namely the humanist notion of the human, and, if possible, contribute to the accelerated transformation of the latter" (Herbrechter 2013: 3). It is "a reflection on how the effects on and of contemporary technoculture and biotechnology force through a rethinking of the integrities and identities of the human: not forgetting, either, those of its non-human others, many of them of humanity's own making and remaking – gods, monsters, animals, machines, systems" (Callus & Herbrechter 2012: 241). Referring to post-structuralist authors like Derrida and Deleuze, some of the more representative authors in this philosophical field challenge the idea of a unified, autonomous subject, thinking on the contrary that this is rather an effect of a complex field of relations, events and structures that it cannot control (Roden 2015). Although the quotation may seem excessively long, precisely because of its relevance for the discourse we will develop later, it is useful to see how Stefan Herbrechter (2013) summarizes some crucial points of the poststructuralist ideas regarding subjectivity and personal identity that he poses somehow as proto-posthumanist:

> "Anthropocentric humanism is first and foremost, of course, human self-representation (cf. Kant's 'What is human?' as the starting point of a (neo)humanist philosophical anthropology). The regime of knowl-edge which accompanies the rise of the humanist paradigm (or 'episteme') within modernity is called 'realism'. Realism is based on the fundamental principles of similarity, the transparency of the medium and of meaningful identity – which means that a situation that was once present, or still is, can, without major loss, endlessly and 'realistically' (that is, true to its reality and originality) be reproduced and thus made present again (re-present-ation). Moreover, this can be reproduced

within any 'subject' who feels individually addressed and who identifies with the reproduced situation, by which it comes into its own, so to speak, and by which it also countersigns the truth of the representation as such. This means that a crisis of realism is also a crisis of its concept of subjectivity. By detracting the subject as 'decentred' – since it is defined both as interchangeable and as uniquely and individually identifiable (i.e., supposed to underwrite the idea of self-identity) – the notion of transparency on which the principle of representation relies also loses its legitimization. Instead, the medium of representation, including symbolic language, of course, develops a dynamic of its own. This, in an extremely simplified form, is the point of departure for so-called poststructuralism: on the one hand, the impossible identity of the subject with itself, on the other hand, Derridean 'différance' at work in symbolic representation, which always promises truth but constantly defers it ('différer', to defer) and therefore always differs from itself ('différer', to differ). The result is a constantly promised but structurally unattainable form of self-identity which conceals or attempts to repress its own difference. Its main 'agent' – the free universal and, at the same time, singular and unique individual – thus exposed or undone, 'liberal humanism' itself becomes incredible as a grand narrative (cf. Lyotard), as ideology (cf. Althusser), as myth (cf. Barthes), or historical and political discourse (cf. Foucault). The most important lever of a poststructuralist critique of humanism is the primacy of language (or the medium, or 'technics' in general) over subjectivity and thus over identity." (S. Herbrechter 2013: 10–11)

2. Transsexualism as an Icon of the Posthuman

Just because of this new way of rethinking human nature, some posthumanist and transhumanist theorists have questioned the role of the body, as a biological *datum*, in determining and/or binding personal identity and sexual gender. In his classic 1950 paper *Computing Machinery and Intelligence*, Alan Turing proposed his famous "imitation game". He invited his readers to imagine being alone in a room, communicating with two entities in another room by two computers. Relying solely on their responses to the questions, they had to decide which was the man and which was the woman.[3] So, paraphrasing Katherine Hayles (1999), it is possible to say that at the inaugural moment of the computer age, the erasure of sexual embodiment is performed so that gender becomes a property of the formal manipulation of symbols rather than enaction in the human lifeworld (Hayles 1999: xi): in effect, in a certain sense, within some posthumanist and transhumanist discourses, the reference to gender, i.e. the cognitive, linguistic and performative aspects of sex identity, seems to erase sex, as a reference for the anatomical, physiological sexual body, and, more specifically, the nature of sexual body as embodied and embedded within the material context. At the same time, transsexualism becomes an emblem of posthumanism/transhumanism, as we think of the ideas that have been developed within these fields, about the subject (identity and its constituents) and the role of technology in relieving modern individuals of the constraints of the body. For example, in her latest book, Rosi Braidotti writes: "what are the consequences of the fact that technological apparatus is no longer sexualized, racialized or naturalized, but rather neutralized as a figure of mixity, hybridity and interconnectiveness, turning transsexuality into a dominant *topos*? If the machine is both self-organizing and transgender, the old organic human body needs to be relocated elsewhere" (Braidotti 2013: 97).[4] Similarly, Donna Haraway (1985), in her seminal paper entitled *A Manifesto for Cyborgs: Science, Technology and Socialist Feminism in the 1980s*, which is an important reference point in transgender theorization, as well as in the debate produced around the theme of the *Post-Human* (Stryker & Whittle 2006: 103, Lechte 2008), like Jean Baudrillard ([1995] 2008), but from a less pessimistic and/or nostalgic point of view,[5] she described the contemporary decline of actually old oppositions of masculine and feminine, along with their corollary distinctions of private versus public, mind versus body, culture versus nature (Felski 1996). She used the figure of the cyborg "in order to [...] imagine a world without gender" (Herbrechter 2013: 100).[6] Martine Rothblatt, from a transhumanistic point of view, stated:

"Advanced technological instruments taught us that people are born with a continuum, not a duality, of sexual biomarkers such as reproductive system morphology, hormonal endocrinology and cerebral neurology. Surgical and pharmaceutical technology enable body-modification into a transgendered realm. Most recently [...] cyber-technology has enabled people to readily clothe themselves in the persona of a limitless variety of sex-types, and to live, work and play online lives in these transgendered identities. Will technology stop at transgenderism? If a century or so of technology has demolished millennia of sexual identity, what might another few decades of exponentially growing technology do? Sex lies at the heart of biology, and yet, in transcending biology, technology gave us an explosion of sexual identities. So, as technology continues to transcend biology, what next can we expect beyond the apartheid of sex? An explosion of human identities? The answer, in a word, is 'transhumanism'". (Rothblatt 2011: para. 8)

3. Beyond/Behind Sexual Identities: Transgenderism and Transsexualism

If we leave apart speculative posthumanism whose main issue is the questioning of future technologically-engendered nonhumans, as hypothetical wide "descendents" of current humans (Roden 2015), at the heart of many critical posthuman/transhuman reflections is the issue of the true nature of subjectivity (Callus & Herbrechter 2012) and the role played by the body and/or other possible non-biological supports for determining/enhancing its qualities. In any case, it is not clear if we are effectively in a post-gender era and how transgenderism, and especially transsexualism, may represent such an instance. Now, two main issues stand out: what is transsexualism and in what way is it different, if at all, from transgenderism? Secondly, how do they come to 'exist'?

The term transgenderism was originally coined by Virginia Prince; it first appeared in a paper of hers in 1978 (Prince 1978) to indicate those men, like herself, who 'elected' to live fulltime and permanently as women, although they were men, without any request for surgical modifications of sexual morphological characteristics. In other words, it was introduced precisely to differentiate such an existential possibility from transsexualism, a term, this, that had been introduced within medical discourse many years before to indicate those who ask for "*sex reassignment surgery*".[7] Now, since the mid-1990s the term transgender has increasingly come to be used as an umbrella term to include different declinations of gender-non-conformity, such as transsexuals, drag kings and drag queens, and so on. Similarly, the latest edition of the *Diagnostic and Statistical Manual of Mental Disorders*, recently edited by the American Psychiatric Association (2013), states: "Transsexual denotes an individual who seeks, or has undergone, a social transition from male to female [MtF] or female to male [FtM], which in many, but not all, cases also involves a somatic transition by cross-sex hormone treatment and genital surgery" (American Psychiatric Association 2013: 451). In any case, although the two conditions tend to overlap, at the same time they seem to differ profoundly. As Rothblatt makes clear, transgenderism may also refer to 'digital gender' subjectivities (Foka & Arvidsson 2014), as subjectivities produced regardless of the specific organic/inorganic support, free from bodily stereotypes. With the support of technical/digital devices, it is said, everyone can shift from one gender to another, or pass as a member of the other gender or any other possible combination of femininity and masculinity. On the other hand, the place occupied by the transsexual is a very different one. As we have already said, transsexual denotes "an individual who seeks, or has undergone, a social transition *from male to female* [MtF] or *female to male* [FtM]." (American Psychiatric Association 2013: 451, our italics) In other words, transsexuals seem to reinforce an *essentialist* position and the *female/male binary*. Moreover, in such a case, the human/material body occupies a special place. To put it better, here it is not the case of subjects who, forgetting their material body, can freely float from one to another virtual universe and "readily clothe themselves in the persona of a limitless variety of sex-types, and to live, work and play online lives in these transgendered identities" (Rothblatt 2011: para. 8). Here, the sexed(modified)-body is the ultimate horizon: it is not the experience of being bodiless or sexless, rather the vengeance of the sexed(modified)-body and, in a certain sense, of the *female/male binary*. Gender is "an identity tenuously constituted in time, instituted on exterior space through a *stylized repetition of acts*" (Butler 1989: 140).

In what follows, we shall initially consider some ideas derived from Jean Paul Sartre's thought with reference to the nature of subjectivity, and in particular of sexual gender, and then propose a critical analysis of the transsexual's condition, starting from the French philosopher's ideas, contrasting them with the posthuman/transhuman theories.

4. Gender Identity and Transsexualism: A Sartrean Point of View

The reference to Jean Paul Sartre's thought may seem at first sight odd if not definitely inappropriate in a discussion of transsexualism as a main *topos* of posthumanism. As we have said before, critical posthumanists, in particular, have accorded special attention to poststructuralist thinkers, such as Derrida, Deleuze, Lyotard, and so on, who tended to see Sartre as a child and a relic of modernity, as a representative of the humanistic and idealistic theories they openly rejected. In any case, over the past twenty-five years, a new critical reading of Sartre has explored the ways in which his and post-structuralist theories interweave and share common ground. For example Christina Howells (1992) has shown how Sartre's philosophical works – from the *Transcendence of the Ego* (1936) to his posthumously published works – prefigure many post-structuralist ideas such as:

"the decentred subject, the rejection of a metaphysics of presence, the critique of bourgeois humanism and individualism, the concept of the reader as producer of the text's multiple meanings, the recognition of language and thought structures as masters rather than mastered in most acts of discourse and thinking, a materialist philosophy of history as detotalized and fragmented." (Howells 1992: 2)[8]

In any case, in our opinion, until now Jean Paul Sartre's original observations with regard to gender identity have not been fully analyzed. Moreover, they may come in very useful for a better understanding of the transsexual condition.

As Sartre states in *The Transcendence of the Ego*, if "The Me (*Moi*) appears through the reflective act and as a noematic correlative of a reflexive intention" (Sartre [1937] 2004: 12), then "the influence of preconceived ideas and social factors, here, becomes preponderant" ([1937] 2004: 16) in determining its 'qualities'.[9] Now, the transsexual issue raises a significant question, when viewed in the light of post-modern thought, about the 'construction' of their personal identity. Stefan Herbrechter stated:

"In a technoscientific culture science is no longer one cultural political component among many, but it becomes the dominant institutionalized economic and ideological power, which fundamentally influences the way people live together, the way they form identities and the forms of embodiment available to individuals, without, of course, necessarily being able to determine these completely." (Herbrechter 2013: 19)

So, considering the infinitely expanding horizontal network of the Web, it is noteworthy to think about the way it contributes to the dissemination of "psychiatric discursive regimes", which, in Sartrean terms, become "preconceived ideas and social factors", i.e. a way to frame subjects' experiences, making them meaningful to themselves and others; in the case of transsexuals', the way such discursive regimes, along with their authoritative and finally explicative powers, enable them to 'interpret' their own identities.[10]

In any case, another question arises: What do we mean exactly when we talk about one's experienced/expressed gender?[11] From our point of view, a good starting point is what Sartre had to say with regard to the differences between the *Real* and the *Imaginary*.

Sartre used the term "real" to indicate the "coefficient of adversity in things" (Sartre [1943] 1956: 392). So, in a certain sense, the anatomy of the body can be referred to this domain. On the other hand, he described the *imaginary* as an attitude of consciousness (Sartre [1940] 2004), which he distinguished from the perceptive domain of consciousness. Perception, he said, is always necessarily *incomplete*, the object never appears except in a series of profiles; imagination, on the contrary, is *total*; imaginary objects – he says – cannot teach us anything, they come from a synthesis of our knowledge and our intention toward them:

> "The image is defined by its intention [...] If the intention is taken at its origin, which is to say when it springs from our spontaneity, it already implies, no matter how naked and bare it may seem, a certain knowledge [...] The intention is defined only by the knowledge since one represents in image only what one knows in some sort of way and, reciprocally, knowledge here is not simply knowledge, it is an act, it is what I want to represent to myself." (Sartre [1940] 2004: 57)

Now, these remarks are quite relevant: whenever we have tried to question transsexual people about what they mean exactly when they refer to their inner feeling of belonging to the opposite sexual gender, somehow they have been surprised, even astonished, by our question and with evident difficulty replied simply offering examples of their favourite activities. But this is not exclusive to transsexual people: after all, for all of us it is extremely difficult to define exactly our being male, female or anything else. Referring to Sartrean thought, our sexual gender appears *total, immediate*. Otherwise, as he said in his *Being and Nothingness*: "Man, it is said, is a sexual being because he possesses a sex. And if the reverse were true? If sex were only the instrument, and, so to speak, the *image* of a fundamental sexuality?" (Sartre [1943] 1956: 383). So, probably, for all of us our gender is similarly developed also on an *imaginary* register, but, in a certain sense, just to say, it is balanced by the *real*, at least by the structure of body, i.e. by the chromosomal sex, the anatomical sex, the reproductive sex and the morphological sex. But this is not enough. Just a little earlier, Sartre had this to say:

> "Of course one may consider that it is contingent for 'human reality' to be specified as 'masculine' or 'feminine'; of course one may say that the problem of sexual differentiation has nothing to do with that of Existence (Existenz) since man and woman equally exist. These reasons are not wholly convincing. That sexual differentiation lies within the domain of facticity we accept without reservation. But does this mean that the For-itself is sexual 'accidentally', by the pure contingency of having this particular body? [...] The fundamental problem of sexuality can therefore be formulated thus: is sexuality a contingent accident

bound to our physiological nature, or is it a necessary structure of being-for-itself-for-others?" (Sartre [1943] 1956: 383)

So, to recap the indications that appear to come from the Sartrean text, gender identity seems to lie somewhere between the facticity of the body, the imaginary and the intersubjective domain.

With reference to the Imaginary domain, returning to the transsexuals' experience, in Sartrean terminology, what they need is an *analogon* – that is, a mental image of femininity/masculinity they conjure when they think of their own possible body transformation. In this sense, the body itself becomes an *analogon* based on "a studied model, reduced to recipes, to schemas" (Sartre [1940] 2004: 27). *Femininity* or *Masculinity* are the signifiers that model the transsexual's body, where this is used, especially in Male-to-Female transsexuals, as a plastic material purposed for continual redesign, in pursuit of a logic guided by subjection to an imaginary ideal of *Femininity* (or *Masculinity*).[12]

For Sartre one can never coincide with oneself because one is always at a distance from oneself. One can never become a *fixed self*, *somebody* in the *substantive* sense. One is always one's *desire*, *lack-of-being*, one's *"possibles"*, rather than an actual entity with substance and structure, a thing (a pure *in-itself*).[13] But, here, in the transsexual case, just to say, "femininity/masculinity become, not always but in many cases, 'master signifiers', *masters* rather than *mastered*.

If it is true that, as Sartre stated in his *Search for a Method*, "language and culture are not inside the individual like stamps registered by his/her nervous system. It is the individual who is inside culture and inside language" (Sartre [1957] 1988: 113), then each of us defines himself/herself as a man or a woman (or anything else), as a *social possible*, according to pre-verbal inner experiences and historical and cultural symbolic references. In such a sense, transsexuals' pre-verbal inner experiences regarding gender identity are signified just within that horizon of meaning opened up by medical discourses, which present themselves as a prominent locus of production for such a "social possible" (Rovatti 2006). More importantly, behind these, they are signified by the *signifier of sexual difference*, which is a culturally and therefore historically determined horizon. It is within this field that we may unequivocally place this "speaking out" about this. In other words, in this case consciousness may direct its own *Ego* as a *noematic correlative*, as a *self-representation*, defining its quality solely and exclusively on the basis of what the social *says* about the *feminine* or the *masculine*.

But this is not all we can say with regard to this condition: As we have seen, Sartre thinks of sexual gender as *a necessary structure of being-for-*

itself-for-others. So, to better understand this existential condition, we also have to consider the importance of intersubjective space.

In his *Being and Nothingness* Sartre begins his discussion of *concrete relations with others* by claiming that we can have two distinct basic attitudes towards another person. In the former, he says, the subject attempts to get the other person to affirm that he does indeed have a fixed nature. He describes this as an attempt to 'assimilate' the other to his project of seeing himself in a certain way. Well, this attitude is clearly evident at least in some transsexual subjects: The significance of the gaze and what occurs in the body image here is quite clear. Within the inter-subjective space, self-mirroring finds a specific eventuality at the worldly level. Now, if in the Sartrean system, the gaze is essentially alienating, the other, at least in *Being and Nothingness*, is seen to represent a necessary threat to one's identity; here we find that, exactly as he states in the chapter entitled *Concrete relations with Others*, the other is often used instrumentally to satisfy the need to confirm one's own existence/self-declaration. It is, indeed, in the gaze of the other that, especially the MtF transsexual, in many cases seeks a prosthetic support, a constant and necessary source of confirmation of her own self-declaration/self-display, and therefore of her own 'assumed identity'. As just a few years ago, the French philosopher and psychologist Patricia Mercader (1994) wrote with regard to the true nature of 'sex reassignment surgery' or hormonal treatments:

> "From a general standpoint, one may wonder whether a morphological transformation can be considered to be a 'sex change': what is trans-formed is the appearance of the body, in other words, the way the individual is perceived and perceives him/herself, the way in which he or she is acknowledged in social life." (Mercader 1994: 18)

Obviously, it is true that for all of us the desire-fuelled gaze of the other is always an important element in defining our own gender iden-tity. To quote Sartre again,

> "My first apprehension of the Other as having a sex does not come when I conclude from the distribution of his hair, from the coarseness of his hands, the sound of his voice, his strength that he is of the mascu-line sex. We are dealing here with derived conclusions which refer to an original state. The first apprehension of the Other's sexuality in so far as it is lived and suffered can be only desire; it is by desiring the Other (or by discovering myself as incapable of desiring him) or by apprehending his desire for me that I discover his being-sexed. Desire

reveals to me simultaneously my being-sexed and his being sexed, my body as sex and his body." (Sartre [1943] 1956: 384)

In any case, what is at stake here, in the transsexual case, is an anthropological lack of proportion: the transsexual individual *ex-sists* her/his own sexual body by erecting it as an index of her/his being within the intersubjective space, as a *plenitude of flesh* often unfurling wholly on the level of the Imaginary. The *irrealizing* action of this register (Sartre [1940] 2004) is, in this case, effectively targeted at the modification of one's own bodily appearance, motivated precisely by the body's nature as a body offered to the gaze.[14]

Evidently, what is achieved through a surgically-modified body, as individuals who undergo such modifications often say, is, finally, the chance to manage to *look-at-oneself* in the mirror, to *find oneself,* to make the reflected image coincide. But, at the same time, a mimetic transformation is also functional to the need to *re-claim oneself* through the gaze of others, the 'imperative' to *find oneself* in the desire-fuelled gaze of the *alter*[15] reduced to a *double reflection*, after the more or less successful cancellation of the last vestiges of ambiguity. Returning once again to Sartre ([1943] 1956), in many cases it is an attempt to use the other "to totalize the detotalized totality which I am, so as to close the open circle, and finally to be my own foundation" ([1943] 1956: 381), a *Perfect, Ideal Woman/Man* beyond *femininity/masculinity* itself.[16] The reconstitution of the image in the mirror, achieved by suppressing male/female bodily signs, therefore finds its deepest motivation in the finally-realized feminization/masculinization of the reflected image, something that initially had only been *glimpsed* in the gaze of others.

What is achieved here closely resembles how Sartre describes the young Gustave Flaubert's experience:

"If Gustave wants to be a woman, it is because his partially feminine sexuality calls out for a change of sex that would allow him the full development of his resources [...] the important thing is that he does not at first designate the recreative valorization of his passivity as a real man, but, on the contrary, as the imaginary woman he wants to be [...] I would say that his first intention is to see himself in his mirror as a woman. Is that impossible? Yes and no; certainly, without faking it, he cannot perceive the reflection of a little girl instead of that of a boy. But – the words 'in order to admire myself' give us a clue – it is possible for him, at the price of a double unrealization, to imagine that he is another who is caressing a real woman, himself, on the far side of the glass [...] There are two analogues here: his hands, his image [...] These two resistances – the reflection, his experienced body – aid him by mutually accusing each another of making the attempt miscarry. If he were completely another, he would be a woman seen in the mirror; therefore, she is there, and to see her he need only unrealize himself a little more. If the reflection would let him become completely feminized, Gustave would be other than the virile hands that stroke him; he would become, there, the absolute object that his caresses here retrieve by internalizing it as excited flesh. A constant and swift passage from one inadequacy to the other will allow him to conceive of the fullness of illusion as accessible and even to imagine, in brief moments of tension, that it is achieved." (Sartre [1971] 1987: 33–42)

Evidently, Flaubert was not in a posthuman era! After all, Sartre himself stated: "the historical whole determines our powers at any given moment, it prescribes their limits in our fields of action and our real future; it conditions our attitude toward the possible and the impossible, the real and the imaginary, what is and what should be, space and time" (Sartre [1952] 1968: 80).

In any case, the transsexual's experience is not easy at all. If it is true that, as Sartre pointed out correctly in his *Being and Nothingness*, "we are always . . . in a state of instability in relation to the Other" (Sartre [1943] 1956: 408), now, in the case of a transsexual, this means that her/his relationship with the other is very, very risky. In fact, the *other-than-Self*'s non-'inert' nature and the individual's dependency on his/her gaze, often makes it a potential source of threat in his/her mind.[17] What is at issue here is that only in a space where she/he is able to see her/his own object-image confirmed that a transsexual seems able to find peace with the *other*; it is only there, in the accommodating gaze of the *alter*, that in many cases her/his anxiety may be assuaged. At least up to a certain point: in fact, their former membership of the male or female gender cannot, for obvious reasons, ever be completely expunged. Vice versa, it will remain as a constantly and potentially re-implementable, *unmaskable* element. A tragic antinomy is therefore set up in such cases on an existential level: if, on the one hand, the other is established as a constant source of threat, on the other, the other's gaze is important for the identity stabilizing process (Vitelli 2015).

5. Some Concluding Remarks on the Relationship between Transsexualism and Posthumanism

Beyond the over-enthusiastic and even triumphalistic tones shown by some posthumanist/transhumanist theorists, as we have tried to show, the transsexual experience may be very difficult. It is not only 'simply' referable to a transcendence of the contingent nature of what is a given in bodily anatomy; to the rising up of an individual above their own facticity through technical advancement. On the contrary, it is a much more complex way of being-in-the-world, in this world! The Biological/Non-Biological, Physical/Immaterial support is not irrelevant at all!

For the most part, transsexuals claim that the mask was the one they were forced to wear before the 'transition' and that what they express, after this transition, is their "true self" (Mason-Schrock 1996). But what is today really a *"true self"*? Without doubt, to some extent, the trans-sexual issue brings with it the need for a more general reflection on the current validity of the ideas produced within the phenomenological-existential theoretical field around the themes of *self* and *authenticity*. Referring to Kenneth Gergen's theoretical considerations, Michael E. Zimmerman stated:

> "In connection with postmodern selfhood, social psychologist Kenneth Gergen has raised two questions: How can one practice being a 'self' at a time when constant change, vastly increased possibilities for relation-ships, transitory commitments, and social fragmentation displace the rational sincerity, integrity, and continuity idealized by the modern self? What does it mean to be a 'self' at a time in which appearances, shifting perspectives, and the infinitely expanding horizontal network of the Web supplant the passionate depths of the romantic self? Although the digitally dominated postmodern age, the once-venerated romantic and modern ideals of authentic selfhood, are being displaced by the 'satu-rated self', Gergen argues that postmodern, decentered, relational selfhood has positive traits worth encouraging." (Zimmerman 2000: 124)

Poststructuralists, as well as many critical posthumanists, have sought to desubjectify or decenter the self, displacing the 'I' from the sovereign role it occupied in modernist theory. They have firmly opposed the self-identical and self-present metaphysical subject. In Lacan's work, for example, the power of the unconscious (in which the 'discourse of the other' is situated) is such that "Man is, from before his birth and beyond his death, taken up in the symbolic chain [...] He is a pawn in the play of the Signifier" (Lacan 1977: 468). The subject, as a site of conscious, autonomous, positive agency, has been, within this philosophical tradition, seriously contested, since it is always constituted within the constraints of institutional/unconscious forces that extend its grasp. As Derrida stated in his *Of Grammatology*, "a self presence [...] has never been given but only dreamed of, and always split, incapable of appearing to itself except as its own disappearance" (Derrida [1967] 1976: 112).

On the contrary, transsexualism seems to remark the opposite. Transsexuals make a strong appeal to *voluntarism*; they affirm that sexual morphology should depend only on *the will of the subject* (Hausman 1999); they imagine themselves as completely *self-transparent* and as completely given in their "conscious appearance". Without any distance from self, rather they claim to re-appropriate themselves, to coincide with themselves; ultimately they affirm the necessity to achieve their "true self". Their place is a far cry from the one claimed for themselves by those transgender people who do not wish to have any somatic transition by cross-sex hormone treatment and/or genital surgery, but do wish to be able to move between the genders. Since the inception of the *queer theory*, and some transhumanistic/posthumanistic stances, there has been great pressure to break down the gender binary system, but many transsexuals do not speak the *queer lexicon* of subverting gender or necessarily identify with the notion of *gender fluidity*.[18] Indeed, transsexual denotes "an individual who seeks, or has undergone, a social transition from *male to female* [MtF] or *female to male* [FtM]" (American Psychiatric Association 2013: 451). In other words, as we have said before, in many cases transsexuals seem to reinforce an *essentialist* position and the female/male binary.

So, might it be that we have to think more appropriately of transsexualism as a response to the posthuman, as an expression of the *old modern ideal of authentic selfhood*? After all, Paula Rabinowitz had this to say:

"Can the posthuman speak? And if so, what's there to say? [...] Speaking is always already something done to us or for us by others whose presence as antecedents, as authorities, as interpreters, overpowers ours [...] Poised between action and representation, posthuman bodies – voguing queens, PWAs – are bodies living outside national, sexual, economic borders. They exceed and override borders by turning bodies into acts and actions into representations. Eliminating the distinction between action and articulation, deed and word, the posthuman body is still saturated with the stories of humanity that circulate around it; it speaks through a language straddling the borders between health/sickness, male/female, real/imaginary. It tells its stories, however, through those already told; it rips off the past to refuse the future. And so the posthuman, alien and marginal like the subaltern, probably cannot speak because it is always spoken through the stories that someone else already told" (Rabinowitz 1995: 97–98).

Notes

1 Some parts of this essay have been published previously in Vitelli (2015).
2 For an historical reconstruction of posthumanism, see Herbrechter 2013; for transhumanistic theory, see Tirosh-Samuelson 2011.
3 In actual fact, Alan Turing posed his famous "imitation game" trying to answer the question whether a machine can think. This is the way Slavoj Žižek summarizes Turing's test: "we communicate with two computer interfaces, asking them any imaginable question: behind one of the interfaces, there is a human person typing the answers, while behind the other, it is a machine. If, based on the answers we get, we cannot tell the intelligent machine from the intelligent human, then, according to Turing, our failure proves that machines can think" (Žižek 2001).
4 In actual fact, Rosi Braidotti's point of view of a transsexual's paradigm has always been much more complex and critical: i.e., see La Fountaine (2008).
5 Baudrillard claimed that ours "is the age of the Transsexual, in which conflicts associated with difference, and even the biological and anatomical signs of difference, continue to perpetuate for a long time after the real alterity of the sexes has disappeared. It is a time when the sexes eye one another up, one through the other. The male eyes up the female; the female eyes up the male. It is no longer a matter of the seductive gaze; it is a generalized sexual squint that reflects the squint of moral and cultural values: the true eyes up the false, the beautiful eyes up the ugly, the good eyes up evil, and vice versa. They all connect, in an attempt to stray from their distinguishing features. In reality, they are accomplices in short-circuiting difference. They act like communicating vessels, in compliance with new machine-like switching rituals. The utopia of sexual difference ends in the switching of the sexual poles and interactive exchange. Instead of the dual relationship, sex becomes a reversible function. In lieu of alterity, an alternating current" (Baudrillard [1995] 2008: 121–122).
6 In 1989 Donna Haraway published *Primate Visions: Gender, Race, and Nature in the World of Modern Science*, her best known work after *Simians, Cyborgs, and Women: The reinvention of Nature* (Haraway 1991). In her own words, most reviews saw this book as being essentially about gender and science, but, Haraway states , "I read the book to be about race, gender, nature, generation, simian doings, and primate sciences. As well as about many other things" (Haraway 2004, cited in Lechte 2008: 334). In any case, with regard to *postgenderism theory*, see Dvorsky and Hughes (2008).
7 For a detailed historical reconstruction of the process of inclusion of the gender variant conditions within medical discourse, see Vitelli (2014).
8 With regard to the similarities and differences between Sartrean thought and Postmodernism, see Fox 2003.

9   In his *The Transcendence of the Ego*, Sartre distinguished an unreflective, impersonal, conscious experience of the intentional objects of those experiences, a consciousness which is ordinarily fully absorbed in the world, coping with the objects around itself, with neither I nor Me, and a "second-degree consciousness" (Sartre [1937] 2004: 58) which grasps the I in its thinking. Only an action of reflection, for the French philosopher, would bring an I "as the unity of actions" ([1937] 2004: 60) and as a self (Me) as a transcendent object. In other words, *selfhood* is only discovered or posited in reflection. More specifically, Sartre distinguishes between two categories of reflected experiences. One of them is that of actions (reflected conscious states in which the self appears as the agent of the action, where the transcendent unity of simple actions is the I, the self as subject), the other one is that of states and qualities, where the self appears as passive. States are, for example, emotional or affective states (for example, hatred which appears in the reflection of the personal conscious experiences of disgust, revulsion and anger). Qualities are in turn that which transcend states, as qualities or dispositions some may say they possess: "failings, virtues, tastes, talents, tendencies, instincts, etc." ([1937] 2004: 16)

10 It is noteworthy that since the origins of humanity the possibility of an area existing beyond the binary subdivision of sexual genders has been incorporated into myth and symbolic representations as expressed through rite, from Plato's Androgyne to Hermaphrodite, from the myth of Attis and Cybele to the figure of Venus Castina. At the same time, different cultures have envisaged, and in some cases continue to envisage, outside any 'pathologized' category, the possibility of there being a non-correspondence between an individual's biological sex and their subjective experience of belonging to a given sexual gender: for example, the 'two-spirits' among American natives, and the Hijras, who still exist on the Indian sub-continent. Nevertheless, in the West today this existential condition is to some extent shaped, and somehow even produced, by a series of discourses, which are first and foremost medical/psychiatric. The transsexual community itself seems to participate in the transmission of master story-patterns derived from such a psychiatric culture which reveal themselves as a way to frame subjects' experience, making it meaningful to themselves and others, and finally to interpret their own identities (Mason-Schrock 1996, Schrock and Reid 2006). With regard to this issue, see also Stone (1991), Billings and Urban (1996).

11 *Transsexualism* can be considered a specific variant of *Gender Dysphoria*, the clinical taxonomic category recently proposed by the American Psychiatric Association (APA 2013). *Gender Dysphoria* more broadly refers to an individual's affective/cognitive discontent with their assigned gender and the distress that may accompany the incongruence between one's experienced or expressed gender and one's assigned gender at birth.

12 One of the people whom Giulia Macoratti, an Italian researcher, inter-viewed a few years ago for an essay of hers had the following to say on the subject: "*The 'top', for a transsexual, is to be Woman, not just a woman … It is what a man sees in a woman … Because [transsexuals] think with*

a man's brain" (Macoratti 2005: 154). In a collection of some autobiographical stories, Porpora Marcasciano, a sociologist and a leading exponent of the Italian transsexual movement, quotes Katy who says: "At that point I told myself that if I had begun the job it would be better to complete it in the best possible way. So, I thought I did well to turn to a good plastic surgeon to tweak my nose, lips, breasts , i.e., fix all those parts that I wanted to be right. In fact, today the work done satisfies me fully: I am the one I had always dreamed of being: the beautiful buxom and buttery blonde Viking! A figure that greatly resembles those women I have always taken as role models for a variety of physical and intellectual qualities. One is Kim Basinger, Nordic, romantic, a dreamer, the *femme fatale* that I have always dreamed of being. I have seen Nine and a Half Weeks time and again, even in slow motion, trying to uncover the secrets of her appeal, to imitate, to reproduce it in my fantasies. Another model of woman that I really like is Alba Parietti, but also Valeria Marini [two famous Italian showgirls and sex-symbols], both considerably surgically retouched, beautifully curvy or, as I say, buttery [...] Let's say that I try to reproduce these models of femininity, a femininity linked to sensuality, the classical charm, a showy femininity . . . in 2006 I had the surgery and I became a woman." (Marcasciano 2008: 80–81).

13 In a very similar vein, from a post-structuralistic/posthumanistic point of view, S. Herbrechter writes "Identity is never identical to itself, but necessarily differs from itself, it is a process, rather than a state" (Herbrechter 2013: 82).

14 For example, Kate Bornstein had this to say on the subject: "I never hated my penis; I hated that it made me a man – *in my own eyes, and in the eyes of others*. For my comfort, I needed a vagina" (Bornstein 1994: 47; our italics).

15 For example, Loredana, a Neapolitan MtF transsexual, had this to say: "I will not deny, however, that working as a prostitute is something we like. It is the desire that we read in the eyes of those men, who, by day, do not look at us and laugh at us, but, at night, belong to us, pay money to have us!" (Cipolla, Rossi, Cardone 2010: 77). Obviously, the issues regarding the transsexuals' prostitution is a much more complex topic. Here we cite Loredana's words just to stress the importance of the 'desire-fuelled gaze of the *alter*' for the identity stabilizing process.

16 It must be said that, for what we have observed in our clinical experience, this is much more evident in MtF subjects than in FtM.

17 For example a subject, quoted by Alessandro Salvini (1999) in a study of his, says this: "*Those who are outside that door waiting to judge me can make me feel like a fully successful woman, or as if I have some original manufacturing defect*" (1999: 260). Furthermore, the sexual encounter itself may be at risk or become a troubling experience: for example, Katy, the person previously mentioned, says: "Sometimes I thought that my partner was staying with me just looking for my male genitalia. This really upset me because I felt like a woman, but if the other was looking for my masculine side, it automatically demolished, cancelled my perception of

myself. This thought was a kind of worm that has gnawed at me for years. It is a problem that I often find myself facing, that the homosexuality of my partner could neutralize my being a woman" (Marcasciano 2008: 81–82).

18 With regard to *gender fluidity* Kate Bornstein had this to say: "If ambiguity is a refusal to fall within a prescribed gender code, then fluidity is the refusal to remain one gender or another. Gender fluidity is the ability to freely and knowingly become one or many of a limitless number of genders, for any length of time, at any rate of change. Gender fluidity recognizes no borders or rules of gender" (Bornstein 1994: 51–52).

Bibliography

American Psychiatric Association 2013: *Diagnostic and Statistical Manual of Mental Disorders. Fifth Edition, DSM-5*. Washington, DC: Author.

Baudrillard, J. [1995] 2008: *The Perfect Crime*, trans. C. Turner. London/New York: Verso.

Billings, D. B., Urban, T. 1996: The Socio-Medical Construction of Transsexualism: An Interpretation and Critique. In R. Ekins and D. King (eds), *Blending Genders: Social Aspects of Cross-dressing and Sex-changing*. New York/London: Routledge, 99–117.

Bornstein, K. 1994: *Gender Outlaw: On Men, Women, and the Rest of Us*. New York/London: Routledge.

Bostrom, N. 2008: Why I Want to Be a Posthuman When I Grow up. In B. Gordijn and R. Chadwick (eds), *Medical Enhancement and Posthumanity*. New York: Springer, 107–36.

Braidotti, R. 2013: *The Posthuman*. Cambridge: Polity Press.

Butler, J. 1989: *Gender Trouble: Feminism and the Subversion of Identity*. New York/London: Routledge.

Callus, I. and Herbrechter, S. 2012: Introduction: Posthumanist Subjectivities, or, Coming after the Subject . . . . *Subjectivity* 5, 241–264. Retrieved November 24, 2015, from http://www.palgrave-journals.com/sub/journal/v5/n3/pdf/sub201217a.pdf.

Cipolla, A., Rossi, L. & Cardone A. 2010: La prostituzione transessuale. In A. Morniroli (ed.), *Vite clandestine: frammenti, racconti e altro sulla prostituzione e la tratta di esseri umani in provincia di Napoli*. Napoli: Gesco Edizioni, 77–94.

Derrida, J. [1967] 1976: *Of Grammatology*, trans. G. Spivak. Baltimore: John Hopkins University Press.

Dvorsky, G. & Hughes, J. 2008: *Postgenderism: Beyond the Gender Binary*. Monographs. Hartford (USA): Institute for Ethics and Emerging Technologies (IEET).. Retrieved November 24, 2015, from http://ieet.org/archive/IEET-03-PostGender.pdf.

Felski, R. 1996: Fin de siècle, Fin du sexe: Transsexuality, Postmodernism, and the Death of History. *New Literary History* 27 (2), 337–349. Reprinted in S. Stryker and S. Whittle (eds), *The Transgender Studies Reader*. New York: Routledge 2006, 565–573.

Foka, A. & Arvidsson, V. 2014: *Digital Gender: A Manifesto – Report on the*

Research Workshop Digital Gender, Theory, Methodology, and Practice (May 15, 2014). Retrieved November 24, 2015, from http://ssrn.com/abstract=2437659 or http://dx.doi.org/10.2139/ssrn.2437659

Fox, N. F. 2003: *The New Sartre: Explorations in Postmodernism*. London: Continuum.

Habermas, J. 2005: *The Future of Human Nature*, trans. W. Rehg *et al*. London: Polity.

Haraway, D. 1985: A Manifesto for Cyborgs: Science, Technology, and Socialist Feminism in the 1980s. *Socialist Review* 15 (2), 65–107. New version printed as A Cyborg Manifesto: Science, Technology, and Socialist-Feminism in the Late Twentieth Century. In *Simians, Cyborgs, and Women: The Reinvention of Nature*. London: Free Association 1991, 149–181.

Haraway, D. 1991: *Simians, Cyborgs, and Women: The Reinvention of Nature*. London: Free Association.

Haraway, D. 2004: Morphing in the Order: Flexible Strategies, Feminist Science Studies, and Primate Revisions. In *Donna Haraway Reader*. New York/London: Routledge, 199–222.

Hausman, B. L. 1999: Virtual Sex, Real Gender: Body and Identity in Transgender Discourse. In M. A. O'Farrell and L. Vallone (eds). *Virtual Gender: Fantasies of Subjectivity and Embodiment*. Ann Arbor (MI): University of Michigan Press, 190–216.

Hayles, N. K. 1999: *How We Became Posthuman: Virtual Bodies in Cybernetics, Literature, and Informatics*. Chicago: The University of Chicago Press.

Herbrechter, S. 2013: *Posthumanism: A Critical Analysis*. London/New York: Bloomsbury Academic.

Howells, C. 1992. Introduction. In C. Howells (ed.). *The Cambridge Companion to Sartre*. Cambridge: Cambridge University Press, 2–9.

Lacan, J. 1977: *Ecrits: A Selection*, trans. A Sheridan. London: Tavistock.

La Fountaine, P. 2008: Deleuze, Feminism, and the New European Union: An interview with Rosi Braidotti. *TRANSIT* 4 (1). Retrieved November 10, 2015 on http://escholarship.org/uc/item/4qf7717m

Lechte, J. 2008: *Fifty Key Contemporary Thinkers: from Structuralism to Post-Humanism* (second Edition). New York/London: Routledge.

Macoratti, G. 2005: Transessuali e transgender: la costruzione di un'identità negata. In C. Fasola (ed.), *L'identità: l'altro come coscienza di sé*. Torino: UTET, 143–58.

Marcasciano, P. 2008: *Favolose narranti: Storie di transessuali*. Roma: Manifestolibri.

Mason-Schrock, D. 1996: Transsexuals' Narrative Construction of the "True Self". *Social Psychology Quarterly* 59 (3), 176–192.

Mercader, P. 1994 : *L'illusion transsexuelle*. Paris: Edition L'Hartmattan.

Prince, V. 1978: The "Transcendents" or "Trans" People. *Transvestia*, 19 (95), 81–92. Reprinted in 2005 in *International Journal of Transgenderism* 8 (4), 39–46.

Rabinowitz, P. 1995: Soft Fictions and Intimate Documents: Can Feminism Be

Posthuman?. In J. Halberstram & I. Livingstone (eds). *Posthuman Bodies*. Bloomington and Indianapolis: Indiana University Press, 97–112

Roden, D. 2015: *Posthuman Life: Philosophy at the Edge of the Human*. New York/London: Routledge.

Rothblatt, M. 2011: *From Transgender to Transhuman: A Manifesto on the Freedom of Form*. USA: Amazon. Kindle Edition, retrieved from http://www.amazon.it/gp/product/B0054SCPKQ?redirect=true&ref_=docs-os-doi_0

Rovatti, P. A. 2006: *La filosofia può curare? La consulenza filosofica in questione*. Milano: Raffaello Cortina Editore.

Salvini, A. 1999: Transessualismo e riorganizzazione della rappresentazione narrativa di sé: un punto di vista clinico. *Rivista di Sessuologia* 23 (3), 257–268.

Sartre, J. P. [1937] 2004: *The Transcendence of the Ego: A sketch for a phenomenological description*, trans. A. Brown. New York/London: Routledge.

Sartre, J. P. [1940] 2004: *The Imaginary: A Phenomenological Psychology of the Imagination*, trans. J. Webber. New York/London: Routledge.

Sartre, J. P. [1943] 1956: *Being and Nothingness*, trans. H. E. Barnes. New York: Philosophical Library.

Sartre, J. P. [1946] 1966: *Existentialism and Humanism*. London: Methuen.

Sartre, J. P. [1952] 1968: *The Communist and Peace*, trans. M. Fletcher and P. Beak. New York: Braziller.

Sartre, J. P. [1957] 1988: *Search for a Method*, trans. H. Barnes. New York: Random House.

Sartre, J. P. [1971] 1987: *The Family Idiot: Gustave Flaubert, 1821–1857 – Volume 2*, trans. C. Cosman. Chicago/London: The University of Chicago Press.

Schrock, D. P. & Reid, L. L. 2006: Transsexuals' Sexual Stories. *Archives of Sexual Behavior* 35 (1), 75–86.

Sorgner, S. L. 2013: *Perfecting Human Beings: from Kant and Nietzsche to Trans- and Posthumanism*. Paper presented at the Fifth International Conference on Kant and Nietzsche, Università del Salento, 18–19 April, Lecce, Italy.

Stone, S. 1991: The Empire Strikes Again: A Posttranssexual Manifesto. In: J. Epstein and K. Straub (eds), *Body Guards: The Cultural Politics of Gender Ambiguity*. New York/London: Routledge, 280–304.

Stryker, S. & Whittle, S. (eds) 2006: *The Transgender Studies Reader*. New York/London: Routledge.

Tirosh-Samuelson, H. 2011: Engaging Transhumanism. In G. R. Hansell and W. Grassie (eds), *H ± Transhumanism and its Critics*. Philadelphia: Metanexus Institute, 19–52.

Turing, A. M. 1950: Computing Machinery and Intelligence. *Mind* 49, 433–460.

Vitelli, R. 2014: Gender Dysphoria in Adults and Adolescents as a Mental Disorder . . . But, what is a Mental Disorder? A Phenomenological/Existential Analysis of a Puzzling Condition. In: B. L. Miller (ed.), *Gender*

Identity: Disorders, Developmental Perspectives and Social Implications. New York: Nova Science Publishers, 55–90.

Vitelli, R. 2015: Adult Male-to-Female Transsexualism: A Clinical Existential-Phenomenological Inquiry. *Journal of Phenomenological Psychology* 46, 33–68.

Zimmerman, M. E. 2000: The End of Authentic Selfhood in the Postmodern Age?. In M. Wrathall and J. Malpas (eds), *Heidegger, Authenticity, and Modernity: Essays in Honor of Hubert L. Dreyfus – Volume 1.* Cambridge (MA): MIT Press, 123–148.

Žižek, S. 2001: No Sex, Please, We're Post-Human! *Lacan.com.* Retrieved November 10, 2015, from http://www.lacan.com/nosex.htm.

CHAPTER
3

Artificial Intelligence and Human Decision Making

SILVIA DELL'ORCO, MAURO MALDONATO, RAFFAELE
SPERANDEO, ROBERTA BARNI, AND LUCOVICA TREMANTE

An increasing amount of scientific evidence in the fields of dynamic systems, statistical learning, development psychobiology and the computational sciences has made obsolete the idea of artificial intelligence and the cognitive sciences that has established itself over the last half century. From the molecular to the social levels, the most highly evolved forms of artificial intelligence are used in discovering the bases of the adaptive flexibility and intelligent behaviour of man. Many maintain that it will not be long before the traditional symbolic-formal domains are supplanted so that it will be possible to set up systems equipped with central control functions, superior cognitive faculties and, therefore, an intelligence able to elaborate abstract-symbolic systems analogous to those of a biological brain. The effect of the advanced hybridization of biology and artificial intelligence, it is believed, might bring into being organisms able to express judgement and take decisions: that is, thinking machines. The birth of such organisms – though having a consciousness not comparable to human consciousness (because incapable of consciousness of consciousness) – might help us to clarify certain aspects of decisional processes that are still little understood, as well as other mental processes that escape our understanding. Considering such a possible future prospect, it is relevant to try to understand the present state of the art relative to (structural and dynamic) problems of (moral) decisions and reduce the doubts that still limit our understanding.

1. A Toolbox of Evolution

The decisional process is an important area of research in the field of artificial intelligence. The ability to take decisions, in fact, is one of the main characteristics of every virtual agent. In general, the latter can choose from a limited number of options. Some of the existing decisional algorithms (Nisan *et al.* 2007) – which enable these virtual agents to choose from a limited number of alternatives – are based on planning, others on reactivity, while still others on a combination of these. In any case, to ensure that the agents take decisions in real time and behave without hesitation, the algorithms need to aim at rapidity and reactivity. This aim is impeded by the fact that the virtual agents are incapable of foreseeing the consequences of a particular behavior. In other words, they do not possess that *toolbox of evolution* (Gigerenzer 2001) which includes intuition, sentience, emotion and heuristics which, since the beginning of time, have enabled man to take rapid and adaptive decisions (Adiandari 2014) and elaborate large quantities of information rapidly and without great cognitive effort.

To have a more precise idea of the challenge, it will be useful to review the empirical research and theoretical positions over recent decades in the field of studies on decisional processes. In the last twenty years, in particular, a large quantity of research on heuristics has shown how impressive is the definition of a more realistic model of the rational agent. The programme of research know as *Heuristics and Biases Approach*, set up in the seventies by Kahneman and Tversky (1973) has made it possible to investigate the limits of the calculation and elaboration of information that leads the individual to adopt heuristics with strong adaptive properties (Kahneman 2011). Heuristics is one of the most effective devices of the human intellect for the reduction of cognitive load and the formulation of quick and generally effective responses to decisional problems (Hamilton & Gifford 1976; Nisbett & Ross 1980). It is a non-deliberate reasoning strategy which allows the individual to choose compatibly with the complexity of the situation and the limitations of his storage and information processing system, by monopolizing normative and probabilistic inferential procedures. According to Kahneman, Slovic and Tversky (1982), heuristic judgement is often the only practical way of evaluating uncertain elements. Contrary to what happens with formal calculation, in fact, heuristic probability assessment is generally based on immediate solutions that do not take into consideration all the factors involved, but only certain aspects: the specific characteristics of the matter being assessed, the formulation of the problem, the clarity with which the situations is described and so on.

Either separately or in combination, these factors influence decisional behavior.

2. Ancient Ecological Wisdom

Over the long process of human evolution, our ancestors have had to adapt to extremely difficult situations. Only quick choices and timely action have ensured their survival. In order to capture a prey moving at high speed, they had to calculate their position in a few split-seconds and be in the exact spot where they prey would be an instant later: a great stress which involved the brain and the whole structure of the body. Not only. It was necessary to get ready for the capture: contract the muscles, overcome the weight resistence and so on (Berthoz 2006). Today, of course, environmental pressures are not what they used to be; but in spite of everything, the brain continues to function in exactly the same way; so we avoid dangerous situations, foresee the intentions of others, and so on. In the light of present-day knowledge, rather than a reactive machine which responds quickly to environmental solicitation, our brain can be described as a proactive machine that enables us to formulate hypotheses, foresee the consequences of our actions, have moves in advance. Difficult adaptive demands have stimulated our superior nervous functions, progressively and as rapidly as possible, to hone the action remodelling capacity of the moment according to unforeseen events. The body itself – the skeleton's architecture, the subtle properties of the sensory receptors, the extraordinary complexity of the central nervous system – has been moulded for the best possible adaptation. These mechanisms have made our brain formulate internal models of the body and of the surrounding world which reflect the laws of nature and enable every animal to survive.

The question of the instant solution to problems – which calls into question the relationship between perception and intuition – was the object of study as early as the first half of the twentieth century of the *Gestalt* psychologists, who showed that, especially in conditions of discrimination uncertainty, perception stratagems closely resemble our intuitive judgements. In fact perceiving means eliminating ambiguities, select one interpretation instead of another: in short, make decisions (Berthoz 2006). And it is thanks to the probabilistic traits of perception that we obtain a uniform representation of our retinal images, which change continually in their shape, size, brightness and other endogenous neurophysiological dynamics. And yet, in spite of these continual changes, our perception of the external world is stable and constant. In conditions of uncertainty, in fact, our perception system, just like our intuitive judgements, "straightens things out" by going beyond the information received: to put it one way, it bets on things being one way rather than another. Think of the phenomenon of "perceptual constancy" (Farah 2000) according to which an object or an event in the surrounding world seems stable and constant in spite of continual external sensory variability. It is this which enables us to perceive the rectangular shape of a door, even if its retinal image varies from one point of view to another. Our brain sees only a rectangle which turns on its hinges, even if when the door is opened it produces a series of trapezoids. It is an energy saving process needed because of the endless demands of perceptual adjustment, which continually prevents risk of inaction. Perceptual constancy also enables us to perceive objects as having unchanging size. In fact, when we see a person or an object in the distance, although the image projected onto the retina is small, we do not have the impression that they are really small in size. They are simply at a distance. This means that, automatically and unconsciously, our brain has compensated for the variations in size of the retinal image caused by variations in distance. Therefore, perception integrates the representation of the physical world, going beyond the information received through continual unconscious inferences (Maldonato 2015a). Every day, we see objects which are partially concealed (a person sitting behind a desk, a dog crouching behind a tree so that we can see only its head and tail and so on), but we perceive them as a whole, so giving a sense to the surrounding environment. In fact, sensory stimuli which are incomplete or devoid of meaning become integrated in the brain with mnenstic or imagined material in order that the whole perception experience is given meaning. This perception, which goes beyond sensory information, is a decision taken by the brain in order to ensure a coherent representation of the world.

3. The Sixth Sense in Action

Intuition is a form of instinctive and unconscious knowledge that allows us – instead of processes of the logical-deductive kind – to look at and deal with issues in a new way, often as if they were already resolved. 'Intuit' (from the Latin *intuèri* – look inside) means looking, getting to know with the mind's eye, which is the most natural, oldest and most universal capacity – a real biological wisdom – belonging to the human being (Mysers 2002). Intuition comes into play in situations when temporal and cognitive-computational bonds prevent us from reflecting on and evaluating the data available to us. It can save us a great deal of effort and is an amazing ally when our survival is threatened. This has been so since the beginning of time: quickly reading the intentions of another increases our chances of survival. This is why the first moments of a meeting may reveal much more than a thousand conversations. After all, in all the cultures of the world the ability to read non-verbal signals has enormous importance. In effect, the great majority of human decisions are intuitive, unconscious and take little psychic effort (Maldonato, Dell'Orco 2011). It is thanks to them that we are able, rapidly and without too much effort, to calculate a considerable quantity of information deposited in our memory, soliciting immediate and often reliable recognition of the present situation on the basis of analogies with past experience, which leads us to new and unexpected solutions to the problems that nag us. Wherever high levels of experience are reached, an incalculable amount of 'visceral' information is accumulated. Think of the chess champion who, after a rapid glance, makes the decisive move, or at least the best possible move at the time; or the expert ento-mologist who easily identifies the class of insect that he happens to come across; or finally, the doctor who, in an emergency, identifies a vital incipient risk in a patient. In every specific field, the ability to distinguish between thousands of possible different situations and objects is one of the fundamental tools of the expert, above all the main source of his intuition (Simon 1983). In the last twenty years, the amount of research on mental instinctive devices has grown significantly and this, as happens in other fields, makes it hard to give a rigorous description.

So what is intuition? Creativity, implicit awareness, implicity learning and memory, sixth sense, heuristics, or emotional intelligence? It's diffi-cult to say. Intuition has characteristics common to these and to other definitions. *Insight*, for example, which is often considered to be synony-mous to intuition, is the sudden understanding of a problem or an solution-finding strategy, an experience of the "eureka!" kind which follows the incubation, mainly unconscious, of a hold-up to the solution of a problem (Oliverio, Maldonato 2014). Intuition takes place almost instantly and is made up of a set of emotional and somatic processes without (at least apparently) rational and conscious thinking playing any role. In fact, intuition almost always as its somatic correlation is accompanied by a sensation in the stomach, a sudden occurrence of thought. But what is the origin of all this? An interesting hypothesis has sometimes been put forward (with a certain metaphysical touch) that there is a crowd of *cognitive workers* (Maldonato 2015b) who, every day, in the underground of our minds and beyond any light of conscious-ness, work on an incredible amount if information that involves implicit memory, heuristics, spontaneous inference, emotions, creativity and much much more. Think of our ability to intuitively recognize a face. Looking at a photo, our brain breaks down visual information into sub-dimensions (colour, depth and shape) and simultaneously elaborates each aspect, comparing the reconstructed image with those which have been sent to memory. Then, immediately and apparently without effort, among thousands of faces we recognize that of a person we have not seen for many years. Of course, this cannot compete with a computer's ability to recognize: the impulses of biological neurons are much slower than silicon neurons. In spite of this, our intuitive and unconscious abilities allow us to work on an incalculable number of actions: catch a ball in flight, convert bi-dimensional images on the retina into tri-dimensional perceptions, tie our shoe laces, make a chess move and an infinite number of other things. Let us look again for a moment at driving a car. We know that learner drivers give all possible attention to driving. They concentrate only on the road. They know perfectly well that they cannot talk to others, and so on. Just the same, with the passing of time and experience, the procedures of driving become automatic and the driver's attention is given to other demanding actions. But things do not always go as they should. Overwhelmed by daily concerns, how often have we returned home without remembering anything about it? And how often have we forgotten to take a motorway exit because we were distracted by a telephone conversations or absorbed by a song on the radio that we have not heard for years? Without any precise indication of a certain destination, our *cognitive workers* automatically carry out the tasks for which they have been trained and that they are used to performing. However it may work, it is thanks to their efficiency that, without effort or conscious control, we can carry out daily tasks and concentrate on what is important.

4. Anticipation, Memory and Action

To act, it is necessary to remember. Memory, however, is not the only device to remind us of past events (both internal and external), but also the whole set of our corporeal perceptions, of the patterns of our sensory-motor habits. There is no paradox in the statement that this contains the possibility of actions which have not yet been performed. Our present is simultaneous sensation and movement. But since they are completely indivisible, movement is dependent on the sensation which extends into action. In this sense, the present constitutes a system made up of sensation and movement: that is, a sensory-motor system. Thanks to the traces of past events lying in our memory, we are able to anticipate future actions by preparing behavior suitable for certain purposes. This is evidence of the importance of a physiology which is proactive in its live and direct relationship with the surrounding environment, compared with traditional reactive physiology. Berthoz (2006) did not advance a paradox when he proposed that there are more than five senses. Many now agree that a perception has various systems of reference modulated by the actions in progress: the receptors measure 'derivates', the brain mobilises a number of prototypes of shapes, faces, objects, and even synergies of movement. In its intricate development, evolution has defined certain simplifying laws of dynamic, geometrical and cinematic properties of natural movements. It is even true that, especially thanks to memory which anticipates the consequences if future action by comparing them with actions of the past, perception shows predictive ability. Through his schema theory (1975), Schmidt has attempted to classify the relationships between perception, action and memory by identifying the relationships between prevision of the consequences of an action and memory of past consequences. His theory is based on two fundamental concepts: generalized motor programming and specific motor schema. The first is a motor pattern held in memory which represents a class of actions with invariant general characteristics. Some of these are: a) the sequence of the muscular contractions of a gesture; b) its temporal structure (that is, the times of realization of single movement segments) which remains constant even with the variation of the overall time of the movement; c) relative force, or the constant proportion between the forces of the various muscles involved, independently of the total force. The variation and adaptation of different situational needs are made possible by changes, during ongoing action, in certain parameters such as the choice if specific muscles and the force and duration of the movement. In sport, for example, the same movement repeated many times will not be identical, even if its basic structures remains unchanged, which confirms the existence of generalised motor programming (Maldonato, Dell'Orco 2012). These variations are made possible by the motor schema, which is a kind of generalisation of concepts (and reactions between them) derives from experience, which enables us to identify what needs to be done in the execution of a motor programme. In other words, while generalised motor programming provides the invariant properties of the desired gesture, the motor schema chooses and adapts the specific parameters of the response to situational needs. Let us suppose that, in order to take a penalty kick a footballer selects a motor programme and calculates contextual information in ways he considers to be most effective. He will adapt the generalised motor programme to that specific situation, modulating the parameters (time of movement, width, position of the foot and so on) to the specific needs of the situation (Schmidt, Wrisbern 2000). The greater the variability experimented on the same motor programme, the more precise the schema. In fact, with each variation of the same class, as with the increase of accuracy in the response feedback, the schema is revised and reinforced as a general rule. In the same way, the elimination of particular information solves the problem deriving from the quantity of data to be stored. Schmidt's schema theory (1975) indentifies two basic aspects: the recall schema, which permits the triggering of new responses and provides the generalised motor programme with the parameters needed in order for the execution of movements appropriate to the task; and the recognition schema, which when the movement is being executed, permits its correctness to be evaluated, comparing sensory feedback in progress with that awaited, so that necessary correction can be made. This is how the sensory consequences if response can be anticipated by comparison, during and/or after the movement, with incoming feedback. In this way, always, information is gathered about the result and any deviation of expected sensory and real consequences recognised. A very similar concept was expressed some time ago by Neisser (1976). He maintains that perception is a 'cycle' whose basic structures consist of anticipatory schema, that is my action programmes which prepare the subject to acquire information which, in its turn, modifies the original schema. In other words, schema is continually modified by experience and the information acquired anticipates future choices. For example, if we carry on one arm a tray of cocktails and lift one to serve someone, we will keep the tray balanced even if the weight on our arm undergoes variation. But if someone takes us by surprise and takes his glass himself, it is certainly less probable that the tray will retain its balance. In this case, in fact, our brain is not able to anticipate the decreased weight of the tray and, an instant before, modulate the muscular tone of our arm. Thus anticipatory modality is based on a motor memory (in this case the reference used by the brain is the horizontal position of the tray in relation to gravity). In the execution of a motor task, the boundaries between perception and action are not so clear as might be thought. One need only consider the calculation ability of the cellular structures, rather than their specific function in carrying out a task, to realise that the role of perception and execution of action is not only that of the frontal lobe, but also of the ganglion cells at the basis of the sequencing of movements, language or ideation (Oliverio 2009). Though parts of different systems, perception and action share the same functions.

5. Moral Decisions: Out of Control?

The complexity and difficulties encountered in the AI research programme were already clear to von Neumann (1958), who clearly
foresaw the obstacles and aporia of a cybernetic model of human
behaviour. Human beings have always been able to solve the issues
that beleaguered them – to distinguish that which is important from
that which is irrelevant, hone their discrimination capacities, be open
to other possible explanations, and so on – as an indirect effect of evolution. The complexity of the issues dealt with shows how extremely
complex is research in the field of decision making. The cultural impact
of AI development is bringing about an individual and collective transformation of humanity. The convergence of AI, genomics and
nanotechnology is opening up possibilities and challenges who for the
moment we can only sense, but not envisage. We are facing a cultural
challenge which will long occupy the minds of those who think that
sooner or later technology will prevail over man and those who believe
in man's ability to take charge of these processes (a large number of the
leaders in the world of production consider moral questions to be in
opposition to progress and innovation and that, because of this, the
rigid predisposition of the moral parameters of robots will keep their
versatility in check). Be that as it may, it is clear that progress in this
field will favour the development of intelligent IT applications which
are able to reason and take moral decisions. AI systems might be used
not only to complement and serve as an addition to human decision-
making processes (providing further information or urging the
decision-maker towards ideas that have been ignored), but above all to
clarify aspects of the complex and, in many ways, obscure dynamics of
decisions.

And then, there is a further matter to consider in relation to decision
making: morals. This specifically human sphere is concerned with
emotion, awareness, the meaning content of information, social attitudes, all that is related to man. Because of the extreme importance of
the issues raised by the supra-rational sphere, the birth of organisms
capable of making decisions poses extremely relevant questions. As has
been ascertained, the emotions play a leading role in the human decision-making process (Damasio 1994, Salovay and Mayer 1990), and
therefore the sphere or moral must have an ontology: a moral decision
is taken, in fact, by human beings wholly immersed in the environment,
their own culture, the relationships they have with others, each with his
own aims, values and desires. Furthermore, in social situations what is
moral is not necessarily predetermined. It is often true that the appro-

priacy of certain actions derives from real situations and precise inter-actions between interested parties.

So that the construction of decisional architectures in hybrid organ-isms or of internal representations of an environment in which every potential action is calculated is very different from the ability to predict the variability and unpredictability of human action. Of course, amazing progress has been made in the development of robots with social abilities (Breazeal 2003), which can learn (Brooks 2002) and which have a theory of mind (Scassellati 2001). However, the possibility of constructing systems able to integrate different skills which might facilitate the devel-opment of higher-order faculties must be relegated to the future. Today's focus on the implementation of competences in hybrid intelligent organ-isms must change to a focus on research into the sphere beyond the ability to reason and decide, above all because of the inevitable implica-tions of consciousness and emotional states. These are inescapable individual and social supra-rational issues which will eventually show the success or otherwise of a path that has been taken on which, to a large extent, depend the fate of humanity as we know it so far.

Bibliography

Adiandari, A. M. 2014: Intuitive Decision Making: The Intuition Concept in Decision Making Process. *International Journal of Business and Behavioral Sciences* 4 (7), 1–11

Berthoz, A. 2006: *Emotion and Reason: The Cognitive Science of Decision Making*, trans. G. Weiss. Oxford: Oxford University Press.

Breazeal, C. 2003: Emotion and Sociable Humanoid Robots. *International Journal of Human-Computer Studies* 59, 119–155.

Brooks, R. A. 2002: *Robot: The Future of Flesh and Machines*. London (UK): Allen Lane.

Damasio, A. 1994: *Descartes' Error. Emotion, Reason, and the Human Brain*. New York: Avon Books.

Farah, M. J. 2000: *The Cognitive Neuroscience of Vision*. Oxford: Blackwell Publishers.

Gigerenzer, G. 2001: The Adaptive Toolbox. In: Gigerenzer G. and Selten R. (eds), *Bounded Rationality: The Adaptive Toolbox*. Cambridge (MA): MIT Press.

Hamilton, D. L. and Gifford, R. K. 1976: Illusory Correlation in Interpersonal Perception: A Cognitive Basis of Stereotypic Judgments. *Journal of Experimental and Social Psychology* 12 (4), 136–149

von Neumann, J. 1958: *The Computer and the Brain*. New Haven/London: Yale University Press.

Kahneman, D. 2011: *Thinking, Fast and Slow*. New York: Farrar, Straus and Giroux.

Kahneman, D., Slovic, P., Tversky, A. 1982: *Judgment under Uncertainty: Heuristics and Biases*. New York: Cambridge University Press.

Kahneman, D., Tversky, A. 1973: On the Psychology of Prediction. *Psychological Review* 80, 237–251.

Maldonato, M. 2015a: *The Archipelago of Consciousness*. Brighton: Sussex Academic Press.

Maldonato, M. 2015b: *Quando decidiamo. Siamo attori consapevoli o macchine biologiche?* Firenze: Giunti.

Maldonato, M., Dell'Orco, S. 2011: *Natural Logic. Exploring decision and intuition*. Brighton: Sussex Academic Press.

Maldonato, M., Dell'Orco, S. 2012: The Predictive Brain. *World Futures. Journal of General Evolution* 68, 381–389.

Myers, D. G. 2002: *Intuition: Its Power and Perils*. London: Yale University Press.

Neisser, U. 1976: *Cognition and Reality*. San Francisco: W. H. Freeman.

Nisan, N., Roughgarden, T., Tardos, Vazirani, V.V. 2007: *Algorithmic Game Theory*. Cambridge: Cambridge University Press.

Nisbett, R. E., Ross, L. 1980: *Human Inference: Strategies and Shortcomings of Social Judgment*. Englewood Cliffs: Prentice-Hall.

Oliverio, A. 2009: *La vita nascosta del cervello*. Firenze: Giunti.

Oliverio, A., Maldonato, M. 2014: The Creative Brain. CogInfoCom, *5th IEEE International Conference on Cognitive Info-communications*, November 5–7, 527–532

Mayer, J. D., Salovey, P. 1993: The Intelligence of Emotional Intelligence. *Intelligence* 17 (4), 433–442.

Salovey, P., Mayer, J. D. 1990: Emotional Intelligence. *Imagination, Cognition, and Personality* 9, 185–211

Scassellati, B. 2001: Investigating Models of Social Development Using a Humanoid Robot. In B. Webb and T. Consi (eds), *Biorobotics*. Cambridge (MA): MIT Press, 145–168

Schmidt, R. A. 1975: A Schema Theory of Discrete Motor Skill Learning. *Psychological Review* 82, 225–260.

Schmidt, R. A., Wrisberg, C. A. 2000: *Motor Learning and Performance* (2nd edition). Champaign (IL): Human Kinetics Publishers.

Simon, H. A. 1983: Alternative Visions of Rationality. In P. K. Moser (ed.), *Rationality in Action: Contemporary Approaches*. Cambridge: Cambridge University Press.

4

On the Relationship between Decision Making and Basal Ganglia: A Computational Perspective

RADWA KHALIL

1. Decision Making and Basal Ganglia (BG) through Computational Lens

Decision making is a crucial high-order cognitive process, which strongly influences everyone's life in different prospective; socially, economically, politically and clinically. Over decades, decision making was (and still is) an interesting topic for the public and the specialists. Therefore, this chapter aims at highlighting several core fundamental questions about the neural basis of decision making from a computational perspective. Basal Ganglia(BG) is thought to be the main gate for controlling and optimizing the decision making through mechanistic interaction with the cortex. Further, several researchers successfully captured the computational features of BG during decision-making process. A connectionist approach is one of the most precise and robust models to reveal the computational properties of the neurobiological architecture during this dynamical process (decision making). This approach enabled neuroscientists to integrate the neural architecture, based on the neurobiological properties, and dynamical features of the particular brain area of interest. Computationally, researchers proved that both BG and Cortex are essential for implementing optimal decision making between alternative actions. Further study illustrated the interaction between cognitive and motor cortico-BG Loops during decision-making process. Focusing on BG, what is its specific functional role during decision-making process? In this context, number of evidences indicated its strong contribution in perceptual decision making (PDM). Since decision making is a dynamical process, which involves competition between cognitive, motor, and limbic cortical and subcortical loops, recent reports implemented dynamical synapses to highlight several aspects underlie synaptic plasticity during the decision-making process such as uncertainty, sequential decision making and reinforcement learning. Despite the great achievements in the field of decision making, in particular PDM, several mechanistic questions are required to be addressed.

2. What do Computational Models tell about Decision-making Mechanisms in the Basal Ganglia (BG) Neural Circuit?

What do the Basal Ganglia do from modeling perspective? (Chakravarthy 2010). This interesting study revealed the functional role of BG computationally. In this study, they designed an architecture of BG. This neural network architecture was representing in seven deep brain nuclei. These nuclei were involved in a variety of several brain functions such as action selection, action gating, reward based learning, motor preparation, timing, etc. Thus, researchers succeeded in providing an integrative and comprehensive view about the functional role of BG assessed to each nuclei.

One successful computational approach for designing BG architecture is the connectionist model due to their fascinating properties. Feldman & Ballard (1982) introduced a connectionist model and their characteristic features, which offered a number of advantages to be applied in cognitive science. For example, it can tackle several critical questions about several dynamical aspects such as stability and noise-sensitivity, distributed decision-making, time and sequence problems, and the representation of several complex concepts. Consequently, further study shaded the light on one of the application of connectionist model as mind architecture reviewing the state of art of such approach (Rumelhart 1989). Moreover, researchers claimed that not only structured probabilistic approaches but rather an integrated connectionist dynamical model enable us to address crucial cognitive questions related to human thought, language, and behavior. On the scope of the application of connectionist approach to address the functional role of BG in decision-making process, number of studies explained the decision-making process in BG through connectionist model (Radwa, K., Martin, G., Andr, G., & Thomas 2013; Martin Guthrie, Charlotte Héricé, Radwa Khalil, Maria Moftah, Thomas Boraud 2014; Héricé, C., Khalil, R., Moftah, M., Boraud, T., Guthrie, M., & Garenne 2015; Charlotte Héricé, Radwa Khalil, Maria Moftah, Thomas Boraud, Martin Guthrie 2016).

3. The Crosstalk between Basal Ganglia (BG) and Cortex to Optimize Choice Selections

Is it possible to optimize the choice selections through BG alone? The answer is no since the crosstalk between both BG and cortex is an essential process to implement the optimal decision making between alternative actions (i.e., action selection) (Bogacz & Gurney 2007). Here, researchers numerated the neuroanatomical and physiological features that relate to the neural circuit of cortex and BG. These biological aspects were essential to implement the computation defined by an asymptotically optimal statistical test for decision making (i.e., the multi-hypothesis sequential probability ratio test (MSPRT)). According to MSPRT (that had been used in this study), cortical mechanisms for decision making were complementary to those in basal ganglia. Therefore, the crosstalk between both brain areas (cortex and BG) is critical for optimized decision making and action selection. Along with the same line, another evidence illustrated the interaction between both cognitive and motor cortico-basal ganglia loops during decision-making process (Guthrie *et al.* 2013). This study was complementary to a previous modeling study by Leblois *et al.* (2006). The model of Leblois addressed a question of how an action selection mechanism in cortico-basal ganglia loops occurs. Therefore, the model of Guthrie went beyond by focusing on describing additional details about the multiple level action selection in BG. The main finding indicated that a decision is taken at the cognitive level, which can be used to bias the decision at the motor level. Additionally, this study highlighted the functional impact of certain neuromodulators during decision-making process.

4. Which Kind of Decision Making could be Performed by BG? Is it a Perceptual Decision Making (PDM)!

We do know that BG is essential for performing decision making. But, what kind of decision making exactly could be taken/performed by BG. Lepora & Gurney (2012) found that BG optimizes decision making over general perceptual hypotheses, which are presented in cortex. Moreover, authors explained this finding in relation to several aspects such as cortical encoding, cortico-basal ganglia anatomy, and finally, reinforcement learning. More insight on the contributive role of BG in perceptual decision making (PDM) was provided by Ding & Gold (2013). This research summarized recent evidences supporting particular computational roles of BG in PDM. Last but not least, Wei *et al.* (2015)

highlighted the functional role of the indirect pathway of BG and beta oscillations during PDM in case of Parkinson disease.

Dynamical Synapses, Spiking Neural Network Models (SNN) and Decision-Making Process

Does decision-making process requires synaptic plasticity? And if yes, then, can we predict its impact artificially? Several studies predicted the influence of synaptic plasticity during decision-making process through implementing dynamical synapses. For example, it was reported the reliability of the synaptic facilitation and neuronal attractor dynamics for sequential decision making (Deco *et al.* 2010).

According to what we previously mentioned through connectionist studies on decision making (Guthrie *et al.* 2013; Leblois *et al.* 2006), the mechanisms of decision making and action selection were gathered to be under the control of parallel cortico-subcortical loops connecting back to distinct areas of cortex through BG and processing motor, cognitive and limbic modalities of decision making. Therefore, recent study by Charlotte Héricé, Radwa Khalil, Marie Moftah, Thomas Boraud, Martin Guthrie (2016) focused on the next step , on the base of these previous findings, toward further development and extension of the connectionist model at a spiking neuron level. This study provided a useful application and great advantage of Spiking Neural Network (SNN) model through linking learning rule to decision-making process in BG neural circuit. For example, authors showed that before learning, synaptic noise is sufficient to drive the decision-making process. On contrast, after learning, the decision turns to be dependent based on the choice (that has proven most likely to be rewarded). Interestingly, this SNN model was then applied to lesion tests, reversal learning and extinction protocols. Under these conditions, it behaved in a consistent manner providing predictions in accordance with observed primates' experimental data.

Conclusion

To sum up, we aimed at providing a brief overview about the influential impact of utilizing the computational approach as a powerful predictive tool in providing a construct about the functional role of BG in decision-making process. Therefore, we provided few examples of relevant research studies as an approval of how and why computational model, in particular connectionist model, can be useful and necessary in revealing the neural circuit architecture underlies decision-making process.

Bibliography

Bogacz, R. & Gurney, K., 2007. The basal ganglia and cortex implement optimal decision making between alternative actions. *Neural Computation*, 19(2), pp. 442–477.

Chakravarthy, V.S., Joseph, D. & Bapi, R.S., 2010. What do the basal ganglia do? A modeling perspective. *Biological Cybernetics*, 103(3), pp. 237–253.

Charlotte Héricé, Radwa Khalil, Maria Moftah, Thomas Boraud, Martin Guthrie, *et al.*, 2016. Decision-making in a neural network model of the basal ganglia. Sixth International Symposium on Biology of Decision Making (SBDM 2016), May 2016, Paris France. <http://Sixth International Symposium on Biology of Decision Making (SBDM)>.

Charlotte Héricé, Radwa Khalil, Marie Moftah, Thomas Boraud, Martin Guthrie, and A.G., 2016. Decision making under uncertainty in a spiking neural network model of the basal ganglia. *Integrative Journal of Neuroscience*, (December).

Deco, G., Rolls, E.T. & Romo, R., 2010. Synaptic dynamics and decision making. *Proc Natl Acad Sci U S A*, 107(16), pp.7545–7549. Available at: http://www.ncbi.nlm.nih.gov/pubmed/20360555%5Cnhttp://www.pnas.or g/content/107/16/7545.full.pdf.

Ding, L. & Gold, J., 2013. The basal ganglia's contributions to perceptual decision making. *Neuron*, 79(4), pp. 640–649.

Feldman, J.A. & Ballard, D.H., 1982. Connectionist models and their properties. *Cognitive Science*, 6(3), pp. 205–254.

Guthrie, M. *et al.*, 2013. Interaction between cognitive and motor cortico-basal ganglia loops during decision making: a computational study. *Journal of neurophysiology*, 109(12), pp.3025–40. Available at: http://www.ncbi.nlm.nih.gov/pubmed/23536713.

Héricé, C., Khalil, R., Moftah, M., Boraud, T., Guthrie, M., & Garenne, A., 2015. Decision making mechanisms in a connectionist model of the basal ganglia. In *The Multi-disciplinary Conference on Reinforcement Learning and Decision Making (RLDM 2015)*.

Leblois, A. *et al.*, 2006. Competition between feedback loops underlies normal and pathological dynamics in the basal ganglia. *The Journal of Neuroscience: The official journal of the Society for Neuroscience*, 26(13), pp. 3567–3583.

Lepora, N.F. & Gurney, K.N., 2012. The basal ganglia optimize decision making over general perceptual hypotheses. *Neural computation*, 24(11), pp. 2924–45. Available at: http://www.ncbi.nlm.nih.gov/pubmed/22920846.

Martin Guthrie, Charlotte Héricé, Radwa Khalil, Maria Moftah, Thomas Boraud, *et al.* ., 2014. Decision making mechanisms in a connectionist model of the basal ganglia. Fourth Symposium on Biology of Decision-Making

(SBDM) 2014, May 2014, Paris, France. <http://sbdm2014.isir.upmc.fr>. <hal-01102619>. *Fourth Symposium on Biology of Decision-Making (SBDM)*, (May), pp. 2–3.

Radwa, K., Martin, G., Andr, G., & Thomas, B. (2013)., 2013. A connectionist approach to decision making in the basal ganglia, p. 1.

Rumelhart, D.E., 1989. The architecture of mind: A connectionist approach. *Foundations of Cognitive Science*, pp. 133–159.

Wei, W., Rubin, J.E. & Wang, X.-J., 2015. Role of the Indirect Pathway of the Basal Ganglia in Perceptual Decision Making. *Journal of Neuroscience*, 35(9), pp. 4052–4064. Available at: http://www.jneurosci.org/cgi/doi/10.1523/JNEUROSCI.3611-14.2015.

CHAPTER 5

The Consciousness of the Inorganic

PAOLO VALERIO AND MAURO MALDONATO

For over a century, the mind sciences have tried to throw light on the most obscure secrets of the brain. But the more maps are drawn, the more mechanisms that are discovered, the harder it becomes to arrive at an understanding. It becomes increasingly clearer that cerebral organization is much more complex and dynamic than was suspected until a few decades ago. Many researchers believe that what will help our understanding of social life will be the powerful development of technology or, more precisely, the face-off between man and computer (of incredible power) which will generate organisms capable of going beyond the simulation of cerebral functions; they will learn from their own inner states, interpret the data of reality, set their own objectives, and converse with humans; above all, they will make decisions on the basis of their own 'value systems'. In a not-too-distant future, it is thought, these organisms will be able to acquire greater and greater autonomy, self-conservation, their own creativity, value hierarchies and, perhaps, even have an ethic based on 'freedom'.

If we are to go far beyond the confines of what today is defined human, to the point of including entities which are the product of hybridization of biological organisms and artificial ones (humanoids, cyborgs and so on), we believe we should consider how we might get there. This is an extremely relevant question which relates to the set of those functions which make man the highest expression of evolution: above all, it concerns consciousness, that huge and complex variety of neurobiological, phenomenological and psychological events that, ever since the first stages of development, have prepared the ground for the emergence of the Self, which enables us to become aware, to lay down values and hierarchies of values, rules and decisions about everything ranging from freedom to necessity.

1. Immaterial Architecture

Although determined by the highest level of cerebral activity, consciousness is inseparable from mental content. It is a complex of distinct material and immaterial characteristics – neural infrastructures, awareness, temporality, qualitative subjectivity, intentionality – so strongly soldered together that they seem to be faces of the same prisma. Consciousness is not a simple function of the mind: it is its very organization. As an expression of distributed neural processes, it does not have a rigid hierarchical order, but is maintained by multiple horizontal levels, each of which is a structural and functional continuum with diverse phenomenal supervenient.

In the course of the centuries, bitter philosophical, religious and scientific controversies have stood in the way of a shared theory, resulting in the consequent fossilization of meanings that have widened its semantic reference, so making the term as polysemous as it is controversial. In fact, the same word is used to describe a spectrum of phenomena which ranges from the most subtle activities of the thought of man to the simple condition of being awake. Until the mid-twentieth century, the idea that biological research could reveal its secrets would not even have been taken into consideration by scientists. After a golden period from the second half of the nineteenth century to the first half of the twentieth – which found its greatest expression in the research of thinkers such as John Hughlings Jackson, William James, Charles Sherrington, Henry Ey, Wilder Penfield, Giuseppe Moruzzi and John C. Eccles – the debate focused, on one side, on the identification of an explanatory model of the ways in which psychological organization generates conscious awareness; on the other, on the understanding of the relationship between neurobiological, cognitive and qualitative processes of experience. Without making any concessions to the arguments of dualists, skeptics and supporters of a materialistic ontology of the 'mental', one relevant position is that of believers in the irreducibility of subjective experience (McGinn 1991). These thinkers, in fact, maintain that our cognitive limitations prevent a clear understanding of consciousness, and therefore, even if we were to discover the biological correlates of our mental experiences, our subjectivity would remain untouched and untouchable. Then there is the position of those who unify cognition and corresponding functional states, putting experience and cognitive behaviour on the same level. It is their belief that the mind and a brain function and mental phenomena (pain, hunger, etc.) should be considered simply from the quantitative, and not qualitative, point of view. For this reason, we need to analyze the modular vertical structures which mediate information exchange between perception organs and central systems which are responsible for more complex activity (Fodor 1983). These modules, each of which is responsible for a specific domain, must be genetically determined and situated in precise cerebral regions. In more radical models, these modules do not exchange information between each other or with central structures, but follow predetermined and unmodifiable computation strategies. From a functionalistic angle, the brain has been described as a multitude of specialized micro-processors distributed and in competition with each other to gain access to a *global workspace* (Baars 1997) of coordination and control of information. Like on a stage with parallel and simultaneous action going on, it is the work of a huge quantity of information below the threshold of consciousness that determines conscious subjectivity. At the basis of such a system there is a thalamocortical circuit which uses its ascendant and discendent projections to give sense to distinct content.

2. The Neurobiology of Consciousness

In the second half of the twentieth century, on the basis of evidence from experiments on the visual system of primates, it was thought that the origin of consciousness was a system mediated by thalamocortical waves similar to that, which presides over the activation of the neurons of certain strata of the visual cortex. Francis Crick (1994) maintained that consciousness comes about in the same way as sight: according to this theory, high visual areas project directly onto the prefrontal areas, creating an intermediary representative space between a lower level of sensation and an upper level of thought. This double dimension is present in the neo-Darwinian hypothesis of Gerald M. Edelman (1989), that there is a *primary consciousness* and a *superior consciousness* which allows the Self to recall and narrate its experiences, freeing the subject from the biological ties of 'here and now'. In this framework, in which the primary consciousness connects the axiological-categorical memory to present perception organization, the upper consciousness operates a synthesis of the value-assessing memory and the categorical memory in the temporal, frontal and parietal areas. From the competition/collaboration between these two neural organizations – the non-Self which is responsible for sensory relations with the world through present experience and the Self which from social relations acquires a meaning and syntactic memory for concepts – we derive artistic ability, ethical systems and a scientific vision of the world. The model of a hierarchical structure of consciousness is more marked in the theory of Antonio Damasio, who thinks that consciousness is indistinguishable from emotion because it derives from a particular physical feeling and consists of various elements: a) a *proto-Self* – based on biological expressions such as fear, hunger, sex, anger and so on – which man shares with higher animals; b) a *nuclear consciousness* which gives the organism a sense of itself, a 'here and now', with no awareness of future; an extended consciousness, which by means of language creates the autobiographical Self (Damasio 1999).

In reality, hierarchically structured models leave many gaps to be explained. How could a schema of this kind deploy dynamic equilibriums among antagonistic organizations (visual, auditory, tactile, proprioceptive and so on) which influence each other reciprocally on the intrasensory and intersensory level to co-determine the content of conscious awareness? What would appear to be more plausible is a dynamic induction model with unity, diversity, variability characteristics, which is integrated into a large neural space (Maldonato 2015). This hypothesizes the work of a set of neurons linked to each other at short distance (but with a certain degree of autonomy) which produce visual, semantic, motor and other phenomena. In this case, the critical role would be played by the frontal lobes and by a distributed aggregate of neurons of the thalamocortical system. In the interface between these structures and the other cerebral areas, there would take place those bioelectrical phenomena with variable and dynamic special distribution, necessary for cerebral integration, differing from one moment to the next, in the same individual and from one individual to another.

3. Intemporality and Duration

By means of consciousness, and differently from the higher animals, humans have developed a capacity of internal representation of time. In humans, this has slowly become consciousness of space. It has taken centuries for time to free itself of its metaphysical identity to become an object of research in the same way as natural phenomena. Modern science has made the distinction between the time of everyday experience and that of religion and philosophy. Up to the beginning of the twentieth century, the psychic formation of space was investigated much more than the psychic formation of time. And yet, while it is true that our experience of time is different from our experience of space, it is not in fact another essence. The sense of time, our experience of time, is a quality of consciousness and as such must be investigated.

Towards the end of the nineteenth century, William James maintained that we can know the phenomena of the mind only in terms of evolutionary adaptation. Our thinking is an expression of a permanent and mutable relation with objects independent of it. James refutes the idea that the elementary data of consciousness are the sensations and that these give rise to levels of awareness which are more and more complex and refined (James 1980). Even an elementary perception is the effect of a subtle abstraction. The *stream of consciousness* describes the passing of thought from one object to another without interruption. No psychological analysis can catch the deep movements of the mind. It is invested not only with ever-moving awareness, but with all that comes in contact with it. In every instant, one or another innumerable processes overlap in our minds, giving is the sense of duration. The most remote moments leave behind them contrails which anchors itself in the present moment. In this *illusory present*, fragments of memory, both near and far, merge with the living present, while the echo of moments which have just gone by resonate in others which are still to come. In this way, time left behind merges with time to come (James 1890). Duration is the name we give to the incessant flow of the past into the future and the future back into the past. Not the sense of before and after. In fact, we are not aware of successive moments. We sense intervals and end-points as one whole. The distinction between beginning and end is an illusion, as is the idea that by paying attention we can separate and distinguish the elements of a perception. The idea of objective time, as an infinite and necessary continuum, is a fallacy. Time cannot be reduced to the causal order of space. The consciousness of time derives from our sense of duration.

There is substantial agreement among present-day researchers that our perception of time derives from the different speeds in the changes perceived in a given period: minimum thresholds of correlation between neural processes and cognitive events indicated by wide-ranging integration and widespread synchrony. But there is no agreement about the nature of phenomena of sequence and duration. For more than a century and a half it has been held that the measure of a period of time between given events is the key to our cognition of time, underestimating the difference between the sequence of neuron events and the order of such a sequence. The occurrence of acts of consciousness is not consciousness of their occurrence. Other models are needed to explain why our states of consciousness are accompanied by the awareness of their occurrence. Acceptable hypotheses about the nature of our perception of sequence and duration indicate the following order: below 100 milliseconds it is possible to distinguish the beginning and end of an instantaneous event; over 5 seconds of perception of duration seems to be halved by memory

(Fraisse 1987). Other authors, such as Francis Crick and Christopher Koch (1992), have postulated as a basis of consciousness a mechanism of temporal standardization of neuron activity which synchronizes medium wave impulses of 40Hz. These waves might not codify additional information, but standardize part of the existing information to a coherent perception. In actual fact, in a further stage of his research Crick threw doubt upon the idea that these waves could be sufficient to generate awareness of an experience, saying that other hypotheses and more complex models of connection were needed.

Apart from the specific frequency of thalamocortical waves, it seems that there are no other doubts about the fact that the origin of consciousness is the simultaneous action of different neuron cortical-subcortical populations and not that of a single cerebral zone. As many electro-encephalographical studies show, there are multiple neuron circuits, activated by parallel synchronization and inhibition phenomena: *transitive states* and *substantive states*, the former activated by a high-energy unstable neuron activity, the latter by a low-energy stable neuron activity. This is a dynamic equilibrium in which each event (an abstract thought, a visual image and so on) reflects the activation of a thalamo-cortical neuron network which produces consciousness content (Le Van Quyen *et al.* 1997).

In discussing consciousness, metaphor is extremely useful. Imagine the brain as being a musical ensemble. As we know, the success of a concert is dependent on the synchronic execution of the instrumentalists of a given score. But how does a score become a tune? A tune is much more than the sum of the notes that make it up. It emerges from the mysterious meeting of frequencies, rhythms, and changes of speed, not from their sum. The combination of the notes of the harps and the piano, the percussion rhythms and so on is very similar to neuron waves, their harmonies and disharmonies. While this model is certainly not sufficient to explain the emergence of subjective awareness, it at least avoids our having to call to our aid metaphysical entities such as the "central theatre", the *homunculus* and so on. This is not implausible as a model of the birth of subjectivity: like in a symphony, neuron evolutions and variations accompany the orchestra without any separate identification.

Relating the issue of consciousness to time would appear to be extremely promising. Time helps us to think more rigorously about definite experimental aspects, such as the significance of using millisecond time scales, which make the oneness of conscious experience nothing more than an illusion. At these levels of time, immediacy vanishes. In fact, there are processes which are apparently irrelevant because they are of infinitesimal duration, which have enormous scientific value. No information can have access to consciousness unless half a second has passed since its arrival in the cerebral cortex.

4. The Sense of Time

In his *Essay on the Immediate Data of Consciousness*, Bergson (2001) compares the specialized view of duration of the positive sciences with subjective duration. Before him, the Greek philosophers, and later Augustine, tried to throw light on the concept of the present, considering time as a succession of present moments. The name he gives to the experience of time – an experience with qualitative, dynamic, discontinuous, asymmetric characteristics – is 'duration'. Bergson maintains that the explanation of time given by physicists is misleading. The purely symbolic time of mathematical equations is an abstraction, a mere sequence of moments placed next to each other; separate segments, identical to each other and indifferent to their content which contrasts with our experience of time, which is duration, change, flux, a continuous and uninterrupted current (Bergson 2001). The key to access to the experience of time, he maintains, is the immediate data of consciousness, the flow of sensations and perceptions that follow one after the other and weave together tirelessly. Subjective time cannot be described as a string of pearls, one next to the other. If any analogy were possible, the only possibility would be the present instant. As soon as it were over, a perception would disappear. We could never experience anything. And if our experience had an order, we could never be aware of it. One idea would follow another. As soon as it were concluded, each state of consciousness would be rapidly extinguished forever.

Many years ago, Schrödinger (1958) observed that physics has no theory that can explain sensations and perceptions. This leads us to suppose that such phenomena cannot be explained by science. At a distance of half a century, it seems even more important to have a physics that recognizes radical differences in time: a physics that first of all would help us to understand how mathematical abstractions, aesthetic preferences, moral judgements and other conscious activities produce dynamics in the brain which are beyond pure computation. But if the mind works in non-computational terms, we must be in a different field from known physics. Roger Penrose (1989) fully grasped this problem, which relates to the radical difference between our perception of the flow of time and the theories of physics. One good reason for believing that consciousness is capable of influencing the judgement of truth in a way which is not algorithmic – notes Penrose – derives from a consideration of Gödel's theorem. If we manage to understand that the role of consciousness is not algorithmic in the formation of mathematical judgement, in which calculation and rigorous proof are fundamental, then we can be convinced that such a non-algorithm might be crucial for the role of consciousness in more general situations (not mathematical). On the other hand, if the functioning of the mind of the mathematician were wholly algorithmic, the algorithm (or formal system) that he himself uses in order to form judgements does not allow him to judge the proposition constructed by means of his personal algorithm (Penrose 1989).

Physics denies that interior time consists of asymmetric moments of duration and intensity. To measure time, it must be spacialized, exteriorized: in other words, it must be expressed in symbols or metaphors such as the movement of the hands of a clock. But clock time is not our experience of time, it does not correspond to that singular and incessant occurrence of thoughts and emotions. The Io manifests its freedom – though still conditioned by and tied to biological bonds – in a movement that rolls out "like that of a thread on a ball, for our past follows us, it swells incessantly with the present that it picks up on its way." (Bergson 1955: 26).

Every experience, every perception, even the most fleeting sensation, is a reflection of living in a continuity, the impression of a permanent flow, not movement from one moment to another. Awareness of time, therefore, is the awareness of an extremely mutable rhythm. The flow of our consciousness has its own endogenous rhythm (liveliness, tiredness, awakeness, sleepiness, dream), varying degrees of clarity, its own specific anomalies and definite pathological expressions. Awareness of an event – an action, a relation and so on, in which something non-cohesive is perceived as a unity – derives from an experience presupposed as being unitary in contrast to the separate moments that make it up, which do not of themselves create the awareness, but grow in it so that it gives rise to its unity. These processes are non-linear, they are part of a multi-level dynamic system which involves complex interactions between brain, body and environment, including conscious and unconscious acts (Thompson, Varela 2001). While it is true that the phenomenon of consciousness is produced by the integrated and distinct activity of the brain, it is at the same time much more. In fact, although it never abandons the body, it goes beyond it to transfigure itself in its individual life separate from environmental events. This fact led Varela to make the provocative claim that "consciousness is not in the head" (Varela 1996) and that the sense of time is an expression of a co-implication of mind and body, not the arithmetical measurement of change. So consciousness is more than its body, something more which does not imply dualism of mind and body, but a unitary and plural experience. This *incarnate consciousness* has temporality as its correlate. A temporality imbued with *intentionality*, the flow of life, which is not synthetic and is therefore temporal; neither synthetic not, at the same time, temporal, but "synthetic because temporal" (Husserl 1991). This is the primary reality – consciousness, in fact – which is always presupposed because its procedure derives from its being *in* time without being *of* time.

5. An Invisible Supremacy

The glow of a firefly, a narrow strip of light, and around it, the deepest obscurity. This is how, more than a century ago, William James described consciousness, that unique psychic faculty – essential to our lives, our thoughts, our image of ourselves – which enables us to understand things in depth, the passage of time, the colours of experience. Consciousness does not impose itself: it is simply present, spontaneous. It is the natural state of things rather than a particular state of things. For a long time it was thought that it was consciousness that allowed reason to guide our choices, our behavior, our reasoning. Today we know that things are very different. Not only do we not know what consciousness is, but we do not even know what it has to do with the world outside us. We know it has a biological function, but we have no idea whether it is the surface effect of a brain which evolved for other purposes. We know only that the awesome number of rational decisions that resulted in that impressive construction which is human consciousness was made possible by a *natural logic* whose laws, most of which are unknown, were extremely useful in evolution.

In any case, even if neurophysiological models appear to be totally insufficient to explain the workings of consciousness, it possesses precise neuronal correlates which have enabled man to develop a kind of *extended adaptivity*. It is therefore inappropriate to state, as some do, that consciousness has a marginal role in human behavior. The latter is exactly what is thought by those who attribute to it an excess of sovereignty in our relational life. Consciousness throws light only on some aspects of our behaviour. It is true that we come up with extremely reasonable explanations on the basis of experience. We distinguish that which is aware from that which is not – a person from a chair, a person who has his wits about him from someone who hasn't – but we underestimate the time for which we are really aware of our actions. Come to think of it, we are not even aware of our unawareness.

To summarize, there are two types of consciousness: the first characterized by qualitative sensations, the second which is without. Despite the fact that perception makes us (qualitatively) aware of objects or facts in the real world does not mean that it is a unique experience. For example, we might be dealing with an abstract problem or a difficult algebraic operation and at the same time aware of it without any specific qualitative or emotional experience. Memories of our lives without any affective resonances are innumerable. But why are some experiences qualitative and others not? That is, how much of us can be considered conscious? We have no idea. All we know is that it enables us to understand our behaviour and adapt it to diverse situations, without ever understanding the multiple essence that makes it up (Bencivenga 2003).

Consciousness is the experience of plurality. But what is plurality? It is certainly not the juxtaposition of entities linked in some way to each other, as if it were a static mosaic. Plurality is the simultaneous existence of subject and object. Without simultaneity consciousness would be unthinkable. And yet, almost paradoxically, for a great part of our daily lives we are absent to ourselves. Think of the *absent presence* we experience during those long car drives we have at least once in a lifetime. Everything rolls past our gaze – landscapes of all kinds, houses, cars going in the opposite direction, clouds of bizarre shape – without our having any consciousness of ourselves. We are one with the car, the road ahead, the landscapes. We drive on for kilometers lost in thought. It is only later that we realize we have driven a long way without realizing it. But what do we mean by "without realizing it"? After all, we have not broken the highway code. Nor have we risked going off the road. Not at all: we have taken difficult turns, without the least hesitation. What was our level of consciousness? Did we take those turns consciously or unconsciously? We may have been aware without realizing it.

On the other hand, if we did not record facts and objects as we drove in this state of automatism, life would be impossible. Our ability to process data and information is drastically limited. And yet mere recording is not enough, just as all possible attention to have full awareness of things and ourselves is not enough. At the most, we unravel fragments of awareness in the darkness of the unconscious. We might even become aware of not being aware, but go on unknowing of the fact that we are in a blind alley, an area inaccessible to thought. And what about consciousness? What role does it play in all this? There is no lack of opportunity: it intervenes in our actions in order to aid their success; it extracts relevant data from the available information so that we can take the best decisions; it analyses the variables at play; it establishes new hierarchies of values, needs and objectives in conflictual' situations; it finds effective solutions to certain problems; and it groups and weighs new and different judgements, drawing conclusions from them.

The multiplicity of levels of consciousness is made possible by a spontaneous order in which the tendency towards oneness alternates with that towards multiplicity. There is no physical-chemical determination, only a flow of processes which has nothing to do with our models or with the terminology we use to describe it: the Io, the Self, the subject, and so on. Clearly this ever-changing scenario brings up the old question of the oneness-plurality of consciousness and how it is able to contain the set of images and emotions related to the body. A monolithic view sees plurality as a sign of retrogression which minimizes the influence of the unconscious universe over conscious life. Awareness and unawareness are not related dialectically, but are deeply involved with each other to the extent of being identical. In the very heart of awareness there are shadows, fantastic refraction, sudden revelations which suggest that it is the Io that makes the decisions, whereas in reality these are elusive happenings which are inaccessible to reason.

Awareness resurfaces every time during the intermittences of thought, in the shadowy states of meditation, during the unexpected flashes of unawareness. There is spontaneous, unexpected and sudden unawareness; as when, during the orderly pauses of our lives, something we did not expect suddenly breaks in, changing the order of things, that stability that we thought we deserved is turned upside-down in the absence of all stability. The ground gives way beneath our feet. We feel as if we are falling. Later, from our regained stability, and remembering that instant – like a kind of *shipwreck with a spectator* (Blumenberg 1985) – we recount that at that moment, as if struck by lightning, we fell. Then there are events that make us unaware in a different way. These events are disturbing, chaotic fantasies that stir our inner being and make us feel life where we are most unaware of being involved in any way: this in the bustle of the body's sensations, in the depths of matter. In this case, it is not awareness of the Io, but something deeper and more indistinct which exists somewhere in the areas where consciousness and unconsciousness interfere with each other. Among these illusory refractions of transparency and opacity, awareness becomes something like the Io in constant changes of perspective. But – and this is a strong but – this is not the Io which is a passive spectator of an imaginary *Cartesian theatre*, but an Io that ascends to the highest levels of an opening to the world of values, laws, decisions, and of freedom. It is *from this point* that thought addresses itself and the things of the world. Not from any abstract point, but a precise *here* (and now) of experience.

6. First or Third Person?

It is almost impossible to talk about consciousness without, briefly at least, mentioning the quality of our experience of the world. For the past half century, this aspect has been at the center of lively debate, above all in philosophical circles. At the heart of the discussion is the concept of *qualia*, the term which philosophers of the mind use to describe perception experiences characterized by the presence of a colour, a sound, a taste and so on. It has been asked: Do *qualia* occur only during emotional states and feelings or also in other states of the mind such as thoughts, enunciations and beliefs? It is undeniable that our thoughts are often pregnant. When we give a cry of joy, of excitement, even ecstatic rapture over the confirmation of a hypothesis, can we really separate ourselves from the quality of the experience? It is anything but a simple realization of a subjectless experience? It is always a first person who experiences something.

How, then, can we understand *qualia*? In two senses, at least: the first relates to the subjective sum of bodily sensations and perceptions; the second, the unintentional properties of certain mental events. From a philosophical point of view, the question has been conceived in relation to the external world. It has been asked, for example, if the behaviour of consciousness and the mind is intentional. Philosophers such as Michael Tye, Fred Dretske, Tim Crane and William G. Lycan have, in different ways, taken up the following position: a mental state, an activity or an internal disposition always have an intention related to an object. A wish is always a wish for something. A thought is always a thought about something. Consciousness is always consciousness of something. So, whether we are talking about perception, or imagination, or thought, the relationship between the Io and objects is always of an intentional nature. The pathway to the *qualia* is such a refined process that it becomes awareness of the awareness of sounds, colours and much more besides. If this were not so, it would be difficult to attribute quality to our experiences. Whatever, we have to ask ourselves whether our mental life relates to objects or to experiences. Because if it relates to objects, it must have a non-relational meaning and the mind must be nothing else but a cold lattice of functionally autonomous nodes. But this is in contrast to the warm and relational idea we have of the mind.

In a well-known article entitled *What Is It Like to Be a Bat?*, Thomas Nagel suggested the impossibility of reducing consciousness to mere neurobiological activity. For this reason, no attempt at naturalization will ever tell us anything about human subjectivity.

Conscious experience is a widespread phenomenon. It occurs at many levels of animal life, though we cannot be sure of its presence in the simpler organisms, and it is very difficult to say in general what provides evidence of it. [...] But no matter how the form may vary, the fact that an organism has conscious experience at all means, basically, that there is something it is like to be that organism. There may be further implications about the form of the experience; there may even (though I doubt it) be implications about the behavior of the organism. But fundamentally an organism has conscious mental states if and only if there is something that it is to be that organism – something it is like for the organism. We may call this the subjective character of experience. It is not captured by any of the familiar, recently devised reductive analyses of the mental, for all of them are logically compatible with its absence. It is not analyzable in terms of any explanatory system of functional states, or intentional states, since these could be ascribed to robots or automata that behaved like people though they experienced nothing [...] I do not deny that conscious mental states and events cause behavior, nor that they may be given functional characterizations. I deny only that this kind of thing exhausts their analysis. Any reductionist program has to be based on an analysis of what is to be reduced. If the analysis leaves something out, the problem will be falsely posed. It is useless to base the defense of materialism on any analysis of mental phenomena that fails to deal explicitly with their subjective character. For there is no reason to suppose that a reduction which seems plausible when no attempt is made to account for consciousness can be extended to include consciousness. Without some idea, therefore, of what the subjective character of experience is, we cannot know what is required of physicalist theory. While an account of the physical basis of mind must explain many things, this appears to be the most difficult. It is impossible to exclude the phenomenological features of experience from a reduction in the same way that one excludes the phenomenal features of an ordinary substance from a physical or chemical reduction of it – namely, by explaining them as effects on the minds of human observers. If physicalism is to be defended, the phenomenological features must themselves be given a physical account. But when we examine their subjective character it seems that such a result is impossible. The reason is that every subjective phenomenon is essentially connected with a single point of view, and it seems inevitable that an objective, physical theory will abandon that point of view (Nagel 1974: 436–437).

Nagel's main question is: What do living beings with sensory apparatus so different from each other as that of man and the bat have in common? Put more simply, what do we have in common with beings different from ourselves? It has to be admitted that we do not yet have a theory and a phenomenology of us and our relationship with ourselves. Only a bat knows how a bat sees the world. With all our minute knowledge of its nervous system, we will never know what kind of experience it has of the world. Having consciousness, Nagel maintains, means feeling to be that particular being: that is, as subject. But if we think about the subjectivity of a bat, it is clear that we shall never know what it feels like to be an individual different from ourselves. This question relates to every sphere of intentionality, and also states such as that of pain – boundary experience between *first person* (the patient's account) and *third person* (biomedical report) – or the condition of patients with great sensory or perceptual impairment (altered states of consciousness, states of minimal consciousness, coma, persistent vegetative state) which we know almost nothing about. How often have we asked ourselves, when the patient is in cold, aseptic intensive care, whether his absence of consciousness has cancelled all trace of subjectivity. Obviously, if we were to adopt the *on/off* model – that is, if tests were concerned only with the defective functioning of awareness – every trace of subjectivity and all conscious content would be cancelled out. But this would only confirm the theory implicit in the premise, without our ever understanding what "Not being conscious" means.

The American philosopher Saul Kripke (2011) claims that pain is only a state of the mind, completely independent of its somatic correlates and different from all other bodily experience or cerebral process. In his view, dualism is fallacious for many reasons. Mind-body identity itself is plausible only in an abstract *possible world*, which would anyway differ from all others, even if in a single detail. In the passage from this world to the other, the definition of entities like mind and body is too rigid. In order to avoid contingency and transience, the mind would have to be identical to cerebral states in every *possible world*. But this is false on the one hand and, on the other, logically impossible (Kripke 1971).

In this debate, the position of the American philosopher Ned Block (1978) is of great interest. He attacks the fundamentalist theory that considers mental events to be similar to algorithms that can be worked out by any machine able to deal with the necessary sequences. According to the believers in *Artificial General Intelligence*, the computer is itself a mind. In fact, if a computer were appropriately programmed, it would not only be able to carry out cognitive tasks, but even be able to understand (other) cognitive states. Block's view is that this is pure conjecture. By means of mental experiments – known as *inverted qualia* and *absent qualia* – he shows how the functionalists are not able even to describe basic experiences such as perception of colour and of pain. A mind, by contrast, is such only because it has qualitative experiences (Block and Fodor 1972). The identification of a mental state with that of a machine presupposes a breakdown of the mind in programmed functional subsets entrusted to *homunculi* with minimal working capacity. But, asks Block, can a set of computerized functions generate the extraordinary diversity of experiences of which a man's mind is capable? Even if it were plausible that these *homunculi* work in the same way as the mind, at the microscopic as well as the macroscopic level, it would turn out to be totally paradoxical.

7. Beyond Human Consciousness

Consciousness is notable for its absence in the scientific research of the twentieth century. But times are changing rapidly. The literature on the subject is growing daily, involving thinkers and researchers in many different disciplines and all over the world. Until now, the Galilean categories have been used in the study of consciousness, those which have enabled us to achieve great success in the explanation of physical phenomena. However, so far these categories have shown themselves to be insufficient in understanding its nature. In fact, no one knows how a physical system (the brain, the nervous system, a set of neurons) can produce that set of phenomena that is our conscious experience. As a result, science does not even know what these phenomena are.

Not even the impressive use of *brain imaging* methods has brought cerebral phenomena to light. As a result, the brain is still a physical object like all the others and we are unable to explain how a certain system can produce conscious experience, whether there is any determinate element which gives birth to consciousness, and finally, whether this develops suddenly or gradually. If science is unable to answer any of these questions, might the way forward be to deal with the problem through the construction of organisms having 'artificial consciousness'? Would it be ethically implausible to try to understand consciousness through refined forms of artificial intelligence?

At the beginning of the third millennium, rather than being able to understand the mind, the decisive act of human history could be made by AI. Until now, we have lacked the technological know-how to construct an artificial conscious being. But now that robots are beginning to resemble human beings – both in terms of computation power and of physical structure – the issue cannot be sidestepped. According to some thinkers, within a few decades the construction of superintelligent machines will enable us to go beyond the human condition (Kurzweil

2005). Left to itself, our biological brain will not be enough. We shall make recourse to nanorobotic systems to help us think, probably by connecting our minds to the *cloud*, the great and potentially infinite store of information on internet. Our very mode of thinking will become a hybrid expression of biological and non-biological elements. As the *cloud* becomes more and more sophisticated, we will upgrade ourselves. With time, the role of non-biological consciousness will become more and more important and consequently our mode of thinking will be more and more non-biological. Once this level has been reached, it is reasonable to think that there will be positive retroaction that will enable the development of further impulses: that is, AI will promote the construction of a better AI, which in its turn will begin the creation of an even better AI, and so on. Regarding the acquisition of new competences by means of self-learning, much will be done to raise this limited intelligence to the standards fixed by machines. It cannot be excluded that a brain capable of extraordinary computation might make possible the development of new senses. It will of course be very difficult to replicate the intricate work of evolution and define sophisticated processing of information as emotions such as pain or pleasure. But it is by no means senseless to think that the speed of technological change will produce such a great impact that it will profoundly change human life: a true discontinuity in the web of human history created by evolution.

Bibliography

Baars, B. J. 1997: *In the Theater of Consciousness: The Workspace of the Mind*. New York: Oxford University Press.

Bencivenga, E. 2003: *Dancing Souls*. Boulder/New York/Oxford: Lexington Books.

Bergson, H. 1955: *An Introduction to Metaphysics*, trans. T. E. Hulme. New York: The Liberal Arts Press.

Bergson, H. 2001: *Time and Free Will: An Essay on the Immediate Data of Consciousness,* trans. F. L. Pogson. Mineola (New York): Dover Publications.

Block, N. 1978: Troubles with Functionalism. *Minnesota Studies in the Philosophy of Science* 9, 261–325.

Blumenberg, H. 1985: *Work on Myth*, trans. R. M. Wallace. Cambridge (MA): MIT Press.

Crick, F. 1994: *The Astonishing Hypothesis: The Scientific Search For The Soul*. New York: Scribner.

Crick, F. and Koch, Ch. 1992: The Problem of Consciousness. *Scientific American*, September, 267(3), 153–159.

Damasio, A. R. 1999: *The Feeling of What Happens: Body and Emotion in the Making of Consciousness*. New York: Harcourt Brace.

Edelman, G. M. 1989: *The Remembered Present: A Biological Theory of Consciousness*. New York: Basic Books.

Fodor, J. A. 1983: *The Modularity of Mind: An Essay on Faculty Psychology*. Cambridge (MA): MIT Press.

Fraisse, P. (1987). Temporal structuration of cognitive processes: Discussion. *Comunicazioni scientifiche di psicologia generale*, 15, 26–33.

Husserl, E. 1991: Lectures on the Phenomenology of the Consciousness of Internal Time. In Id., *On the Phenomenology of the Consciousness of Internal Time (1893–1917)*, trans. J. Barnett Brough. Dodrecht/Boston /Kluwer. Kluwer, 3–137.

James, W. 1890: *The Principles of Psychology*. New York: Dover.

Kripke, S. A. 1971: Identity and Necessity. In M. K. Munitz (ed.), *Identity and Individuation*. New York: New York University Press, 135–164.

Kripke, S. A. 2011: *Collected Papers Vol. I*. Oxford: Oxford University Press.

Kurzweil, R. 2013: *How to Create a Mind: The Secret of Human Thought Revealed*. New York: Viking Press.

Le Van Quyen, M., Adam, C., Lachaux, J-P., Martinerie, J., Baulac, M., Renault, B., Varela, F. J. 1997: Temporal Patterns in Human Epileptic Activity Are Modulated by Perceptual Discriminations. *NeuroReport* 8, 1703–1710.

Maldonato, M. 2015: *The Archipelago of Consciousness: The Invisible Sovereignty of Life*. Brighton/Chicago/Toronto: Sussex Academic Press.

McGinn, C. 1991: *The Problem of Consciousness*. Oxford: Blackwell.

Nagel, Th. 1974: What Is It Like to Be a Bat? *Philosophical Review* 83, 435–450.

Penrose, R. 1989: *The Emperor's New Mind: Concerning Computers, Minds, and the Laws of Physics*. Oxford: Oxford University Press.

Schrödinger, E. 1958: *Mind and Matter*. Cambridge: Cambridge University Press.

Thompson, E. and Varela, F. J. 2001: Radical Embodiment: Neural Dynamics and Consciousness. *Trends in Cognitive Sciences* 5, 418–425.

Varela, F. J. 1996: Neurophenomenology: A Methodological Remedy for the Hard Problem. *Journal of Consciousness Studies* 3 (4), 330–350.

6

The Acceptability of the Artificial: The Attitude toward Post-human

Daniela Conti, Alessandro Di Nuovo and
Santo F. Di Nuovo

In this chapter we will summarize studies about the attitudes and acceptance of artificial life and post-human robotics. Recent technology advances and research achievements boosted the area of robotics that has seen a fast growth of possible applications with concrete impact on the everyday life of the common people. But are these technological forms of 'humanity' acceptable for humans?

1. Fears and Prejudices about Post-human Robots

The users, individuals and operators, need to be helped to have a more realistic view of the advantages and limitations of artificial life and robotics, in order to avoid both a prejudicial refusal and a similarly uncritical enthusiasm.

As regards the first aspect, the *Eurobarometer* survey (2012) reported a generalized distrust for the use of robots in education and health assistance. This reflects a general fear toward robots, well exemplified by the famous movie *2001: A Space Odyssey*, where Hal 9000, a computer "incapable of making mistakes", that recognizes and evaluates ideas and emotions, is ready to kill humans when he thought it necessary to serve what he considered essential goals.

The risk that intelligent machines can rebel, taking over humans, is replicated in the *Terminator* saga where androids, robots and *cyborg* (cybernetic or bionic organisms) are created by the supercomputer *Skynet*, endowed with artificial intelligence, which acquires self-consciousness aimed at taking power by destroying the human race.

Resuming the taboo stated in the fiction novels of the *Cycle of Dune*, after that in the past the thinking machines had been able to enslave humanity, the use of artificial intelligence is even forbidden: the first commandment of the religion of the new empire was: "Machines similar to the human mind have never to be built".

The risk that fictions and movies tell, regards perhaps the danger of a specific artificial intelligence, which does not reflect the genuinely human intelligence. The intelligent machine, when searching for a solution to a problem, scans quickly all possible combinations, as endowed of a "theoretical intelligence".

On the contrary, the "practical intelligence" that is used in everyday life, do not always evaluate all the possibilities and heuristics, but select some of them according to different reasons (time available, accessibility of elements for the solution, interests, motivations, emotions), as studies on problem solving and decision making have clearly demonstrated.

This is the reason for which many users fear that machines become substitutes for socialization and treatment with children and adult persons, "de-personalizing" and de-vitalizing education and rehabilitation (Wolbring, Yumakulov 2014).

Artificial intelligence, to have ecological validity, should represent *practical*, not only *theoretical* intelligence. But in what extent can we simulate desire or apathy, or fulfilment tension, selfishness or empathy: that is, all the motivations related to emotions which constitute the actually implemented human intelligence? These components should be simulated not only in algorithmic way, but also with regard to the multiple and variable adaptive or maladaptive effects dependent on a variable and unpredictable context.

The artificial intelligence can be useful – for its speed and efficiency of calculation – as a support to integrate the concrete intelligence: i.e., when it is useful to consider all the alternatives for achieving adaptive behaviours, compensating for the motivational or emotional deficiencies that inhibit the real person to weigh all the variables in an algorithmic way. But the artificial intelligence becomes useless, or even harmful, if simulates a reality that does not match that of humans, and wants even impose it, because programmed to this end: coming to plan the destruction of humans – as in many movies and fictions – if not fit perfectly rational purposes and means.

2. Too Much Trust in Artificial Technologies?

Surely, we have to cope with negative attitudes and fears toward the artificial lives; but we have also – on the other side of extreme attitudes – to avoid the attribution to them of competencies that are outside of their real possibilities. Sophisticated systems, like *Siri* intelligent assistant for *iPhone* and *iPad*, use attractive user interfaces in natural language to answer questions, give advice, and take action by means of web services, adapting flexibly to the demands and offering highly personalized answers. Many people use these advanced technologies or widespread *chatbot*, always available on a cell phone, as companions to overcome moments of solitude, as friends who make up the feeling that "no one (human) listen to us".

The wish to establish relations without the risk of emotional troubles or possible disappointments, having a partner always available, leads many teenagers and adults to invest in artificial supports altering the very notion of humanity. They develop toward simulations an attitude of confidence, trust and positive affectivity that replace difficult and complicated relations with humans. In the relationship with an artificial agent the emotions are simplified, and the person is less subject to the vulnerability; people will expect more by technology than by humans (Turkle 2009, 2012).

People – especially children and elderly – can increase their sense of attachment also for simple domestic automata, and the risks associated with more socially engaging robots, used to help people in need of assistance in the field of mental health, deserve further experimental and clinic attention and research. In fact, the risks associated with robots that are being used to help people address sensitive mental healthcare needs are not well understood (Rabbitt, Kazdin, Scassellati 2014).

In considering the expansion of Social Assistive Robotics in mental health care, people who are in regular contact with robots are likely to get emotionally attached to these machines. Addressing the concern of the relationship and breakdown of that begins with transparency about the possibility of technological problems and shortcomings, so that users should not be shocked if they occur (Kalvi Foundation 2012).

3. Post-humans in the School

Among the applications of Artificial Intelligence and robotics in social contexts, those regarding education and care of children have received more attention, due to uncertain experimental evidence and the ethical problems more frequent in education.

Benitti (2012) reviewed the scientific literature on the use of robotics in schools and suggested that educational robotics can act as an element that enhances learning, if appropriately used. Several studies have also demonstrated a positive impact of robotic platforms on typically developing children as teaching assistants (Mubin *et al.* 2013). In particular robotic assistants have the potential to overcome concerns about the physical effects of children's use of computer-based tools (Dockrell, Earle, Galvin 2010), because they encourage children to be mobile during a game (e.g., Tanaka *et al.* 2006). As an example, Fridin and Belokopytov (2014b) show that preschool children interact more with a robot than with a virtual agent when involved in a motor task. The robot in the classroom can be a practical learning partner that motivates students in learning and elicits learning performance naturally (Chang, Lee, Wang, Chen 2010).

A robot can be a useful companion and assist a teacher to provide a constructive learning experience supported by several senses: visual, auditory, and touch (Fridin 2014). Robots create opportunities not only to learn from a non-threatening, three-dimensional inanimate object, but also to learn through interaction with other human beings, thus encouraging autonomous social behaviour. This has enabled robots to fulfil a variety of human-like functions, as well as to aid with the goal of improving social skills in individuals with disability (see chapter 1).

Despite the scientific success and increasing evidence and applications, it seems that the majority of people is still sceptical or even contrary to the application of robots in real contexts like education and care of children.

According to Eurobarometer (2012) survey, the European respondents have a general positive attitude towards robots, but 60 percent of them say that robots should be banned out from the area of child, the elderly and disabled care. Furthermore, only 3 percent say that robots in education are a priority, while 34 percent specifically state that are against their use (i.e., they should be banned) in education. This is related to the common perception of robots as *impersonal* and potentially *dangerous* machines, which are mainly useful in space exploration, in military applications and in industry, where there are no human beings around or just the ones that are employed to control them. The survey was very general and participants were given only very limited information about the concept of robots and how they could be used; therefore the responses reflect stereotypes more than real knowledge about the object to be evaluated. However, this negative attitude toward using artificial entities in the care of humans is one of the biggest challenges that scientific research in robotics must address to be successful in giving actual benefits in the field of children's education and therapy.

To fill the gap between stereotypes and real knowledge there have been many studies on the factors that can influence the acceptance by potential users and on how it can be increased. Among the objectives of current robotics research is the adaptation of the robot appearance and behaviors in order to improve the acceptance by the user (Broadbent, Stafford, MacDonald 2009; Kanda, Miyashita, Osada, Haikawa Ishiguro, 2008).

The factors that influence the acceptance of Information and Communication Technology by school teachers have been reviewed by Buabeng-Andoh (2012), that identified several personal, institutional, and technological issues that limit the adoption and integration of these technologies in teaching and learning. Robots were not explicitly discussed in the review. Indeed the researches about acceptance of robotics have often regarded older people in assisted living scenarios (e.g. Broekens, Heerink, Rosendal 2009; Chen, Chan 2011; Klamer, Ben Allouch 2010; Smarr *et al.* 2012), but relatively few studies have been conducted with other participants such as children or their educators and caregivers.

In general robots' acceptance by younger children is difficult to assess because it is not possible to reliably administer the common questionnaires, thus acceptance factors are indirectly derived observing the interaction (Salter, Werry, Michaud 2008).

School children's perceptions and evaluations of different robot designs were studied by Woods (2006). A sample of children evaluated 40 robot images and judged human-like robots as aggressive, but human-machine robots as friendly. This result on children's perceptions of the robots' behavioural intentions provided tentative empirical support for the *Uncanny Valley*, hypothesized by Mori, MacDorman, Kageki (2012): the more the artificial organism is similar to human body, but without reaching the perfect likeness that is typical of video games or movies, the more it arouses fear and reduces acceptance. If an android robot looks indistinguishable from humans, but its behavioural skills are limited and do not correspond to what we can expect from a being with the same appearance and ability as humans, then feelings of repulsion and eeriness can be experienced.

As regards teachers, a recent study (Fridin, Belokopytov 2014a) presented a first attempt to examine the acceptance of a humanoid robot by a group of 18 preschool and elementary school teacher, showing a good attitude and intention to use.

Another study (Conti *et al.* 2015) reported the results of a study on robotics acceptance by a group of 55 students in psychological and educational sciences, and 25 practitioners specialized in the education and care of children with special needs. The reliability of the models of acceptability (e.g., Fridin 2014) was confirmed in the context of education and care of children; all participants, when informed about the use and possibilities of social assistive robotics, showed a positive attitude toward them. The comparison between the two groups highlighted that some scepticism remains among the practitioners, while students show an overall positive perception and significantly higher willingness to use the robot. The result is due not only to differences in age, but to the professional experience of the practitioners that allows them to identify practical issues that could be encountered in the use of a robot with children affected by severe intellectual disabilities.

The literature permit to conclude that the Socially Assistive Robotics is currently perceived by practitioners as a tool, although expensive and often limited, which may provide a real advancement over the other established techniques only if more synergistically integrated with standard protocols and constantly supervised by an experienced professional.

Future work is needed to investigate the acceptance in a cross-cultural dimension. People with different nationalities tend to rate their experiences with robots differently on usefulness, enjoyment, sociability, anthropomorphism, and perceived behavioral control (Eurobarometer 2012; Li, Rau, Li 2010), because each culture has its own level of exposure to robots through either media or personal experiences (Broadbent, Stafford, MacDonald 2009). Studies aimed at extending the sample with students (Conti, Cattani, Di Nuovo, Di Nuovo 2015) and practitioners of different nationalities could assess the impact of culture on the results.

A general conclusion about the acceptance of the post-human artificial organism is that it can never be taken for granted, but it should be analyzed case by case. The acceptability of new technologies based on simulation and robotics by the users and their families but also by the professionals has to be tested specifically before beginning the use: it cannot be assumed that the technologies are effective 'in itself', forgetting necessary mediation of users' attitude and motivation.

4. The Ethics of the Artificial

Researches on acceptability of the practical applications of human–robot interaction, particularly with children or elderly or disabled users, propose more general issues pertaining to ethics. A more careful consideration of the legal, medical and socio-ethical use of the artificial life is needed.

Van Wynsberghe (2014) examined the ethical implications of robots for the treatment and care of elderly and unhealthy persons, proposing a framework for action in which robot designers must be explicit about the values, customs, and contexts of use. A direct dialogue with all communities and users involved in the use of the artificial life appears necessary. In particular, in the context of robotic applications for assisting patients and the elderly, the main recommendation is to empower all users (professionals, patients and/or families) to maintain full responsibility of the care, rather than delegate it to the technologies.

A proper consideration of the ethical aspects of artificial life, especially in child-robot interaction, should lead to a close collaboration with experts from the social sciences like as developmental and social psychology, in order to shed light on the correct and ethical use of the technologies.

Attitudes and perceptions of the users have to be taken into account before and during the interactions between human and artificial, to make these relations suitable and fruitful in the specific context where they are implemented.

Bibliography

Benitti, F. B. V. 2012: Exploring the Educational Potential of Robotics in Schools: A Systematic Review. *Computers & Education* 58 (3), 978–988.

Broadbent, E., Stafford, R., MacDonald, B. 2009: Acceptance of Healthcare Robots for the Older Population: Review and Future Directions. *International Journal of Social Robotics* 1(4), 319–330.

Broekens, J., Heerink, M., Rosendal, H. 2009: Assistive Social Robots in Elderly Care: A Review. *Gerontechnology* 8 (2), 94–103.

Buabeng-Andoh, C. 2012: Factors Influencing Teachers' Adoption and Integration of Information and Communication Technology into Teaching: A Review of the Literature. *Journal of Education and Development Using ICT* 8 (1), 136–155.

Chang, C. W., Lee, J. H., Wang, C. Y., Chen, G. D. 2010: Improving the Authentic Learning Experience by Integrating Robots into the Mixed-reality Environment. *Computers & Education* 55 (4), 1572–1578.

Chen, K., Chan, H. S. 2011: A Review of Technology Acceptance by Older Adults. *Gerontechnology* 10 (1), 1–12.

Conti D., Cattani A., Di Nuovo S., Di Nuovo A. 2015: A Cross-cultural Study of Acceptance and Use of Robotics by Future Psychology Practitioners. *IEEE RO-MAN The 24th International Symposium on Robot and Human Interactive Communication,* 555–560.

Conti, D., Di Nuovo, S., Buono, S., Di Nuovo, A. 2016: Robots in Education and Care of Children with Special Needs: A Study on Acceptance by Experienced and Future Professionals. *International Journal of Social Robotics,* 1–12.

Dockrell, S., Earle, D., Galvin, R. 2010: Computer-related Posture and Discomfort in Primary School Children: The Effects of a School-based Ergonomic Intervention. *Computers and Education 55*, 276–284.

Eurobarometer 2012: *Public Attitudes towards Robots*, Special n. 382. European Commission.

Fridin, M. 2014. Storytelling by a Kindergarten Social Assistive Robot: A Tool for Constructive Learning in Preschool Education. *Computers and Education 70*, 53–64.

Fridin, M., Belokopytov, M. 2014a: Acceptance of Socially Assistive Humanoid Robot by Preschool and Elementary School Teachers. *Computers in Human Behavior 33*, 23–31.

Fridin, M., Belokopytov, M. 2014b: Embodied Robot versus Virtual Agent: Involvement of Preschool Children in Motor Task Performance. *International Journal of Human-Computer Interaction 30* (6), 459–469.

Kalvi Foundation 2012: *Recipe for a Robot: What It Takes to Make a Social Robot*. Retrieved from the Kalvi Foundation website: http://www.kalvifoundation.org/science-spotlights/ucsd-recipe-social- robot.

Kanda, T., Miyashita, T., Osada, T., Haikawa, Y., Ishiguro, H. 2008: Analysis of Humanoid Appearances in Human–robot Interaction. *Robotics, IEEE Transactions on 24* (3), 725–735.

Klamer, T., Ben Allouch, S. 2010: Acceptance and Use of a Social Robot by Elderly Users in a Domestic Environment. *Pervasive Computing Technologies for Healthcare (PervasiveHealth), 2010 4th International Conference*. IEEE, 1–8.

Li, D., Rau, P., Li, Y. 2010: A Cross-cultural Study: Effect of Robot Appearance and Task. *International Journal of Social Robotics 2*, 175–186.

Mori, M., MacDorman, K. F., Kageki, N. 2012: The Uncanny Valley. *IEEE Robotics and Automation Magazine 19*, 98–100.

Mubin, O., Stevens, C. J., Shahid, S., Mahmud, A. Al, Dong, J.-J. 2013: A Review of the Applicability of Robots in Education. *Technology for Education and Learning 1* (1): 209–15.

Rabbitt, S. M., Kazdin, A. E., Scassellati, B. 2014: Integrating Socially Assistive Robotics into Mental Healthcare Interventions: Applications and Recommendations for Expanded Use. *Clinical Psychology Review 35*, 35–46.

Salter, T., Werry, I., Michaud, F. 2008: Going into the Wild in Child-robot Interaction Studies: Issues in Social Robotic Development. *Intelligent Service Robotics 1* (2), 93–108.

Smarr, C.-A., Prakash, A., Beer, J. M., Mitzner, T. L., Kemp, C. C., Rogers, W. A. 2012: Older Adults' Preferences for and Acceptance of Robot Assistance for Everyday Living Tasks. *Proceedings of the Human Factors and Ergonomics Society Annual Meeting 56*, 153–157.

Turkle, S. 2009: *Simulation and its Discontents*, Cambridge/London: MIT Press.

Turkle, S. 2012: *Alone Together: Why We Expect More from Technology and Less from Each Other*. New York: Basic Books.

van Wynsberghe, A. 2014: *Robots in Healthcare: Design, Development and Implementation*. Farnham: Ashgate.

Woods, S. 2006: Exploring the Design Space of Robots: Children's Perspectives. *Interacting with Computers* 18, 1390–1418.

Wolbring, G., Yumakulov, S. 2014: Social Robots: Views of Staff of a Disability Service Organization. *International Journal of Social Robotics* 6, 457–468.

CHAPTER 7

The Force of the Affections: The Becoming-body, the Becoming-free

ROSELLA CORDA

The Posthuman is currently the most ambitious and complex class of anthropological studies because of the diversity of disciplines it includes and the number of attempts at synthesis that have been made of them. This shows that this field of epistemology is significantly close to the Schelerian idea of philosophical anthropology which focused on embracing all the results of sciences having man as their object of study in order to obtain an overall picture in tune with the times, given that never before – and in this sense we can continue to consider ourselves Schelerian – the man would be so problematic for himself (Scheler 1926 and 1928).

This essay assumes that anthropo-de-centralism, the hetero-referentiality of possible co-evolutions (with the earthsphere first and the technosphere later), excess despite biological deficiency (Marchesini 2002), are necessary components of the posthuman paradigm, and will discuss some thematic passages pertaining to the thought of the French philosopher Deleuze, although he does not deal with the topic explicitly.

The condition of possibility of a critically open anthropological profile offered by the posthuman – where the prefix 'post' is intended to point to the critical nature of the matter in question rather than give an exhaustive definition covering a series of multidisciplinary observations – is here interpreted in the light of Deleuze's thinking in his references to Nietzsche and Spinoza.

Revisiting the themes of what Deleuzean literature calls the "great Spinoza-Nietzsche identity" (Fadini 1993, Zaoui 1995) will show the condition-possibility of a posthuman profile in the relationship between the plane of immanence and the affections, in the sign of a "synthetic constructivism"; it will be alternative to the inhumanism characterizing the crisis of the twentieth century subject, and able to increase a bio-techno-anthropological project where the human dimension appears in the powerful virtuality of its hetero-references which are always active from the beginning. The body, or rather becoming-body, is an open field in which the posthuman subject is able to constitute itself in all its singularity. Consequently, starting from the "ground of the affections" concept driven by Spinoza, Nietzsche and Deleuze, and from the radical empiricism emerging from the categorization of the plane of immanence implicit in our topic, we shall examine the meaning of the fundamental anthropological question "What is man?" in the sense of "What can a body do?" as we work towards a rework hinging on the originally and constitutively affective dimension of the human. A new anthropological image cannot emerge except on the basis of a reflection which, in terms of open constructivism, covers the relationship between the question "What can a body do?" and the question regarding the feeling. Critical reflexivity marked by sentiment as the dynamic element of self-diagnostic motivation (how I feel) is to be understood as a radical tonalization of a posthuman horizon whose conservation, in mutation (Masullo 2008), cannot neglect the affections as indispensible "biological sentinels" (Damasio 2003). The freedom *of* the posthuman, at this point, will be found in the singular condition of creative reflexivity in the light of necessary and substantial relationality, in accordance with the model developed by the authors.

The plane of immanence defined as chaosmos is theorized by Deleuze in the development of his thought from a particular type of empiricism whose origin is in Hume's work (Deleuze 1991) in which criticism of the modern subject – and of Kantian transcendentalism – was done through a re-elaboration of the ideas of the British thinker based on his particular view of the open construction of the human mind as a "collection without an album". However, for a true Deleuzean elaboration of transcendental empiricism meant in terms of a special affective tonalization, pared down to its essentials and therefore of high theoretical resolution as a plural analytic (microphysics) of forces, reference must be made to the exegetic relationship with the mediator Nietzsche (Deleuze 1983), and the way of using the integrated philosophical perspective of Spinoza. The synthesis produced by this (Deleuze 1994) reveals the fundamental category of the plane of immanence as a "complex topology" able to produce increasingly new conditions of thought – concept constructivism (Deleuze/Guattari 1994) – and just as able to promote a new post-metaphysical ontology where every form of ontological and essential "eminence" is removed *ab origine* (Deleuze 1994). Deleuzean (and Guattarian) geo-philosophy introduces coordinates whose valence inevitably erodes the traditional position of the ontological-metaphysical question "What is the being?"

(reformulated, especially in modern times, in nihilistic key, in terms of "Why is there something rather than nothing?") in order to radically redirect its formulation, as question of the problematic, to an ontological and epistemological *fold* in which the sides are no longer recognizable in the opposites potency/act, but virtual/actual (where the logical-possible is the opposite of the real).

Returning to the discussion on Nietzschean themes starting from *Difference and Repetition* (Deleuze 1994), a few years after his 1962 monograph *Nietzsche and Philosophy* (Deleuze 1983), Deleuze relaunched the idea of the centrality of an appropriate reinterpretation of the German philosopher's philosophy in spite of traditional reading proposed by Heidegger (1979 and 1984). The real issue at stake is not to be found in a hermeneutical quibble as much as in the possibility of precluding or not the use of critical tools capable of taking into consideration key aspects of contemporaneity: in other words, a new image of thought. For Deleuze it would be insufficient to oppose the Same to the Identical for the purposes of a suitable thought of the original difference and so withdraw it from mediation, and that the Heidegger's criticism to the Nietzsche's Eternal Return would deny the very effectiveness of its effort to conceive the being substracted from all subordination to the identity of the representation (Deleuze 1994). It is well known as Heidegger relegates Nietzsche in the "fulfillment of metaphysics" category of modern nihilism, the definitive strengthening of the absolute modern *subjectum* of which the Will to Power is the ultimate expression. Without in any way going beyond the traditional metaphysical question about the essence of being in general, Nietzsche would replied with the notion of Will to Power, proposing this as *essentia* and consequently the Eternal Return of the Same as *exsistentia*: that is, if the basic assumption is Will to Power as will to overcome in the sense of proposing the being of the entity as the value and therefore as condition of conservation and growth of life (which would be again Will to Power), then what returns is the Same. It is in this way, then, that strengthening/fulfillment of the *identical* comes about, in a will to know folded into being as presence, and resolved in the representation of a substantial subject. This dynamic is at the very basis of Heidegger's philosophy of technology, which sees the contemporary technological dimension, the age of technology, as "oblivion of being" that leads the entity to the annihilation. From the analysis of the moral aspect of Nietzsche's metaphysics (the essence of Being as value given that essential Will to Power would be the principle of the new position of values) emerges the nihilist mould of his thought. And it is noted that Heidegger, who also provides a great stimulus to a profound rethinking of an appropriate interpretation of a new thought, proposes nothing other than a 'poetic' reading of the issue: focus on Being, authentically, starting from Being (*Seinsfrage*) and not from the entity. The thought of the Difference, properly understood and claimed for itself, would replace the repetition of the same, with the ontological fold of the *Selfsame* in the *Aletheia*.

Deleuze's interpretation is different; his interest in Nietzsche is not in the surreptitious introduction of a metaphysical question (What is entity). Having tacitly oriented himself towards a criticism of representational metaphysics in the above-mentioned monograph on Hume, he moves away from the groundwork of empiricism, understood as active experimentation. The idea of subjectivity changed radically its substance, becoming the critical problem of specific human nature, that is of *how the subject is constituted*. Subjectivity came to be understood as procedures *in progress*, movement-mutation, which takes shape as it *improves itself and reflects on itself* in the Hume sense of the activity of *inference, invention, belief* and *artifice*. The idea of a neo-constructivism of the subject, in the form of an open structure, already appeared similar to the Nietzschean characters of a *becoming subject*. The problem of human nature was posed almost according to a genealogical logic, that is, how the principles (which are the reason of its formation) were instead become.

The really new aspect of Deleuze's reading of Nietzsche is in its recognition to the author of *Zarathustra* a fierce criticism to the negative through the logic of affirmation, which gives rise to an original ethic perspective. *Meaning* and *value* are the key terms which appear in the opening of the 1962 work and *genealogical evaluation is totally* focused on the dynamic and differential concept of *force*, split itself as multiplicity (not as separateness). If Kant has recognized the Copernican revolution of the anti-dogmatic act of transition from the essence to the phenomenon and therefore to the examination of the criticism and the centrality of the question of the subject (human), to Nietzsche is ascribed the radical breakup of the gesture. If the question of sense appears in Kant, the introduction of value creates a radicalization. Criticism is carried out "with hammer strokes" (Nietzsche 2008), so nothing concerned may be spared. The *a priori* is returned from the universal to the point of view of approval and the typological and topological question is asked. From "What is it?" to "Who?", in a movement of anti-dialectical immanence. The transition to the value is explained with the idea of Will to Power understood as a genealogy of strength, and from here we are taken to the overthrow of Nietzsche's idea which from the western centrality of the logos moves to the centrality of the body. The Strength is the dynamic and pathic element of bodies.

According to Deleuze, Nietzsche aims to hit the *indifferential* assumption that connotes the traditional idea of origin (or causal derivation) and foundation, for which the values would be indifferent to its origin, or the origin indifferent to values. By introducing genealogy as the value of origin and the origin of value, it affirms the overriding differential internal relation, immanent, *of* and *between* centers of variable forces; force itself is to be understood as the intimate multiplicity of an origin always at plural: the genealogical seed. In fact, only force may have itself as object and enter essentially into a non-mediated relation with itself, involving the Difference – as a potential difference – to realize this own relation.

This differential, relational and immediately pluralistic original complexity is called hierarchy. Relation and hierarchy are not to be understood in the dialectical sense, but in a precise and extremely meaningful aspect depending on the role played by the negative. The aversion to the radical negative is the theme of Nietzsche's anti-dialectic – assuming, that is, that dialectic means presupposing a certain form of negative. Strictly speaking, interpreting Deleuze exegete of Nietzsche, it should be stated that rather than a form of anti-dialectic, this is an hyper-dialectic or post-dialectic. In other words, we should not oppose the dialectic, but oppose that dialectic which nourishes itself of negative, and take charge, perhaps, of an alternative and differential, dialectical logic. The negative, in this sense, is present, but as total active aggression of affirmation.

The *indifferent* element of the philosophy, what is worth in itself and for all, is the universal element. Starting from the *point of view of appreciation* is to accept the evaluation as *ways of being*, singular, freed from the genealogist. *Indifference*, therefore, is replaced by *the pathos of distance, in* and *of difference*. *Genealogical criticism*, in the redundancy of the formula, refers to the total positivity of the *activity* of creation. The introduction of meaning (sense) and value means accepting, once and for all, that it is always a question of making the *difference*: difference, which make the evaluations on the basis of certain values and difference, which make certain values on the basis of the evaluations that presuppose them – and above all, therefore, the difference that *is made* as the fount: disparity, imbalance, partiality and positive detraction, arrest and unavoidable innovation.

The meaning of a phenomenon, then, is given by the strength that takes possession of it. The question itself about meaning is diagnostic and not metaphysical: in place of "What is it?", which presupposes a traditionally metaphysical essence, we have "What meaning does it have?", and ultimately "Who?" This position makes stronger the correlation between meaning and phenomenon (replacing both the dualism appearance-essence and the mechanical relation cause–effect), in a synthetic constructivism: if the meaning of a phenomenon depends on its strength (*which possesses it because it is not separated from it*), it is clear that its meaning is a "complex notion" because that force is a concept which refers to a dynamism. To evaluate is to diagnose: it unravels dynamisms and it is in its turn the effect of an unravelling of dynamisms.

Will does not indicate an action over something which is presupposed, but over another will. Nothing which is representational has yet been described about this and this resolution of thought. The dynamism does not come about between will and something of another nature (as if we radically changed the resolution of an image), but always between a *qualia* of will and another one: between a will which 'orders' and one which 'obeys'. Both these wills are such and they want, but they want with a different intensity. There is no relationship between voluntary and involuntary but between different intensities of strength and therefore, more subtly, of will. "Thus pluralism finds its immediate corroboration and its chosen ground in the philosophy of the will" (Deleuze 1983: 7). Hierarchy is the configuration of the dynamism of will as strength split and taken on by genealogy, and it is the same with the issue of "free spirits", or rather how the conditions of freedom can be provided or if *freedom is the condition of every making-free*.

The hierarchy, it is said, is not understood in dialectical sense – or pyramid – thanks to how the differential element replaces the negative determining it as a *product*: "The negative is not present in the essence as that from which force draws its activity: on the contrary it is a result of activity, of the existence of an active force and the affirmation of its difference [...] For the speculative element of negation, opposition or contradiction Nietzsche substitutes the practical element of *difference*, the object of affirmation and enjoyment. It is in this sense that there is a Nietzschean empiricism" (Deleuze 1983: 9).

Since *The Birth of Tragedy* (Nietzsche 1994), the negative coefficient in the "tragic" would be in the sense of an identification of differential and not dialectical kind. In appearance contradictory, Nietzsche presents himself as a thinker of total affirmation, of the *Ja sagen*, and at the same time as *the first man who finds out the nature of tragedy*. This double-sidedness, however, is to be understood as a strong *trait d'union* between affirmation and tragic thought. The figure of Dionysus in ancient Greek tragedy is symptomatic, characterized as the divinity who shows the suffering instead of 'solve' it. The pain of life cannot be mediated and, more profoundly, there is no contradiction between suffering and life. The tragic cannot be a negative indicator of any opposition. The tragic man is he who says yes to life and has no need to justify his suffering. Pure affirmation, pluralism and essence of the tragic say the same thing: *individuation*. The full positive of *individuation*. Excess: a distributed and scattered fullness as in the dismemberment/laceration of Dionysus. Only a pure affirmation is able to take care of the individuation of every single life. Suffering life – *wanting* from a carence – which should be redeemed, is instead taken to be *fullness* able to deliver itself from all evil. Not only evil is not the rebuttal of life; life, because of its excess, *justifies* the suffering of which it is the healthy carrier. This is the real tragedy. Evil and the negative seem to be functional to the economy of salvation through a designated eminence – and not the opposite. The outward appearance of affirmation says of the further-excess of the *N*-individuated: yet another profile of a disrupted, immeasurable series. The idea of evil weakens in affirmation, losing its meaning. And the tragic is tied to affirmation because only full affirmation sup-*ports* life, admitting a radical tragedy without the option of any cathartic mediation.

In order to express the tragic, however, we have to call into play an affection as its emblematic condition of endurance: joy. This corresponds to that dimension of 'fullness' which gives the affirmative coefficient able to offer life in its total innocence: a condition which allows to integrate the partial integrity of life (its differential matrix). While pain, the *topos* of philosophical literature as the elective place of the drawing out of a genuine dimension, triggers mechanisms of dialectical resentment nourished by the negative and source of further negativity, only joy can be considered a condition of affirmative and non-reactive assumption. The essence of the tragic is "multiplicity, in the diversity of affirmation *as such*. What defines the tragic is the joy of multiplicity, plural joy. This joy is not the result of a sublimation, a purging, a compensation, a resignation or a reconciliation [...] *The tragic* is the aesthetic form of joy, not a medical phrase or a moral solution to pain, fear or pity" (Deleuze 1983: 17). If the essence of the tragic is in the multiplicity which springs from pure affirmation, the joy in which it finds expression is clearly not the effect of a catharsis: a liberation from the negative. It is not a dialectical affection: it is an *expressive* affection in the Spinozian sense. The logic that responds to this affective tonalization is the same as that which gives life to the logic of "typing" in contrast to *exemplum*. Aesthetics and expression indicate the same exclusive level of the problem, radical empiricism, in accordance with the following characteristics: the affective tonalization in discourse (reference to the *value of the affections* as the original condition), the affective tonality specifically chosen (joy), the *expression* of the affective architecture described (the affections *express*).

The question of meaning and value intercepts the existential question as *the most empirical and 'experimental' of problems*. Radical empiricism, in fact, does not dismiss the question about existence, although it doesn't ask about it as an anguished corollary of the Leibnizian question *why is there something rather than nothing*. One might imagine a solution in the name of an indifferent nonsense, but even here there is a good case for a question of difference. If existence has a sense or not, we need to ask, given our premises, not where to place the eminence from which it would derive a liberating absolution (or even libertarian, in the killing of the father who does not kill but reinforces the "interior fascisms", so strengthening the Oedipus guilt mechanism – Deleuze/Guattari 2003) but the strength (of will) which ignites it and favours its creativity. We must look into ways of liberating creativity at the same time as thinking of new forms of life; *experimental* ways of subjectivation which presuppose a tragic freedom of field, where the subject exists in the "one dies" of its caesura of immanence, so postulating the need of a creative liberation of "poietic" energies in the name of a full affirmation. It was said that evil *belongs* to life. It cannot be *abstracted* from it and therefore become its opposite, understood as an objection which should give rise to a question which, being about nothing at all, ends in a negative freedom: freeing itself as it relieving itself from evil – where "itself" coincides with the object of a substantially negative anthropology. If life has a meaning, it intercepts the question of justice but not in the sense of a pyramidal-based justice: a tribunal of conviction or absolution. Full difference does not sway like a pendulum between reclusion and absolution – trained by other interventions. Difference is a movement of radical freedom caught in the lens of transcendental empiricism: *the empiricism of the principles that they have become*. Rather, affirming empiricism and affirming the positivity of freedom is the affirmation (throw) of the *only throw of the dice*.

Difference does not exist between two presupposed elements: difference is the creation of elements. These do not pre-exist but they befit themselves. To assume that elements are in themselves separate, within which to establish a hierarchy or a hierarchical difference, means abstracting these elements by an artificial, or at least tendentious, metaphysical process of injecting the negative factor. It is at this point that the elements become reciprocally distinct but, substantially, indifferent and therefore it becomes possible to swing in inertia between two options. Where, on the contrary, it is wholly a question of *evaluation and difference*, there is always the creative newness of the co-individuated elements. The meaning of existence, then, plays as strength and tension of will (of power) starting from a radical differential-virtual freedom and with a view to a making-free of actual-fact in individuated forms of life. Hierarchy and justice, with a new meaning, are understood to be the same, so breaking down the door of the temple of the Kronos empire, remaining on the threshold of *Aion*. Neither *hybris* nor guilt. Innocence is the sum of existence that finds its way as a joyful expression of a form of creative life. Innocence responds as necessarily conditioned to the freedom as a condition – in the "crack" of the subject. Existence is just in so far as it is innocent. Innocent means *irresponsible*, where responsibility is a feedback retracing the rings of the knots of essence-appearance and/or cause/effect. Irresponsible means "fullness". The becoming (of which existence is the expression) is just in the sense of this innocence. The injustice of time is based on the positing of counterfactual incompossible series of events, *separating the force from that which is in its power*. The series of controfactuals are assigned virtually and not like in a sequence of opposition possible-real (*aut-aut*). The opposition possible(logical)-real separates force from what is in its power in an abstraction that distorts its meaning: "We create grotesque representations of force and will, we separate force from what it can do, setting it up in ourselves as 'worthy' because it holds back from what it cannot do, but as 'blameworthy' in the thing where it manifests precisely the force that it has. We split the will in two, inventing a neutral subject endowed with free will to which we give the capacity to act and refrain from action" (Deleuze 1983: 23). In this case, writes Deleuze in accord with Nietzsche, we are "bad players", to use the metaphor of the "bet".

To propose the difference (with its distances and subtractions) instead of the separateness (and its mystifications) corresponds to the same operation of affirmation of becoming, which demolishes all thinking focused on the negative – that same thought that is unable to understand the concept of tragic. *Hybris* is opposed to the game: "It is not guilty pride but the ceaselessly reawoken instinct of the game which calls forth new worlds" and Deleuze continues: "Not a theodicy but a cosmodicy, not a sum of injustices to be expiated but justice as the law of this world; not *hybris* but play, innocence" (Deleuze 1983: 25).

The metaphor of the dice game, which consists of two moments (the throw, as abandonment to life, and the fall, as a reflection on it), indicates the knot that holds together chance and necessity, chaos and cosmos. The Eternal Return of the Same is their *synthesis*. The combination produced by chance is necessary: chance affirms necessity because the logical possible, which would preclude the necessariness of the necessary, is pure mystification. In the *chaosmos* it is not possible to win or lose: to bet entirely means 'win' but outside the dialectic-hence without any awards. The alternative is not like the abyss of the *aut-aut*: no combinatory could have been different – therefore stands out as necessary. It is only in the *indifference* of a retrospective abstraction that we can measure the equidistance of combinations assumed as possible options. The one throw of the dice puts everything into play, offering itself as a (necessary) repetition of difference. The "good player", the *fuoriclasse* (literally: out-category, or in French: *hors pair*), is he who can think of taking the greatest risk; his position is beyond all victory and defeat: it is an incomparable, new, creative combination. The necessity expressed by chance, its fate, rewrites the rules of every assignment of value: whether an event is a 'victory' or a 'defeat'. The "bad player", on the contrary, throws the dice many times, presuming he can govern, thus, the process of causality and probability, in the attempt to achieve the combination initially declared, by assigning a purpose to the game. The "reason-spider" hatches the plot-web, so "to abolish chance by holding it in the grip of causality and finality, to count on the repetition of throws rather than affirming chance, to anticipate a result instead of affirming necessity – these are all the operations of a bad player. They have their root in reason, but what is the root of reason? The spirit of revenge, nothing but the spirit of revenge, the spider. *Ressentiment* in the repetition of throws, bad conscience in the belief in a purpose. But, in this way, all that will ever be obtained are more or less probable relative numbers.". Conversely: "that the universe has no purpose, that it has no end to hope for any more than it has causes to be known – this is the certainty necessary to play well. The dicethrow fails because chance has not been affirmed enough in one throw" (Deleuze 1983: 27).

This complex affective condition of the *fuoriclasse* can be traced to he who, in his last work, Deleuze calls the "exhausted" (Deleuze 1995), in contrast to the "tired". While the tired is he who is bowed down by not being able to realize any possible, the exhausted is he who can no longer possibilitate: "The tired can no longer realize, but the exhausted can no longer possibilitate" (Deleuze 1995: 3). The impossibility of possible, the zeroing of certainties and options of choice is the only situation in which one *can* have the affirmative epiphany, and so enjoy the fullness of a joy of the warrior. The affirmative attitude of the *fuoriclasse* is desire and he invests himself completely; he does not desire in the grip of lack, anticipating another dimension at which to aim, but he has complete faith in "*amor fati*" – or he throws himself "headlong", as Deleuze and Guattari write more soberly of Kafka (Deleuze/Guattari 2003): absolute risk is to a desire that loves, betting entirely. Fatal affirmation has two interrelated affects: joy and love. *Amor fati* is the essential obliteration of the tragic.

"Universal chaos which excluded all purposeful activity does not contradict the idea of the cycle; for this idea is only an irrational necessity" (Deleuze 1983: 28): chaos and cycle have always been seen as opposing and alterative elements in that, as seems obvious, the cycle indicates an ordered repetition which excludes chaos. The cycle would impose a curve on chaos, tightening it into the rigid belt of *logos*. When this happens, rationalizing and measuring chaos in the cycle of a return (that is, within a repetition whose form is generality), chaos is lost; conversely, if we fail in the task of imposing a curve, we escape into a chaos where all possibility of equilibrium is frustrated. The 'final' return, the eschatological fold of time, puts the chaos of the becoming under constant threat: either one genuflects in the presence of the end and of the purpose, finding a definitive order, or one goes mad. In the extract from Nietzsche mentioned above, a different attempt at synthesis is proposed: the necessity that alone can bend chaos without distorting its creative potential is irrational, as long as the connotation of irrational does not enter into the dialectic of the rational. Irrational must be understood as being an indication of creativity, or of incommensurability. To affirm the chaos of the becoming is to affirm the return. The return is the unity (the *identity*) of the becoming. Thinking pure affirmation is thinking the completely *new*. Citing a passage from *Zarathustra*, Deleuze concludes: "Will, this is what the liberator and the messenger of joy is called" (Deleuze 1983: 36, Nietzsche 2006: 110).

There is another ambiguity to clear up. The double affirmation and its necessity cannot evade the dimension of "must-be". Not at all: it is because of the double affirmation that this "must-be" seems in its chronogenesis to be more terrible. This is not a "must-be" which has developed on the basis of a metaphysical adequacy which requires a moral mould: it is rather a complete giving over to the dimension which is more properly and poietically ethical.

Returning to the comparison with the Thinker of the *oblivion of Being*, we can now come to a conclusion about exactly how alternative the Deleuzian exegetic perspective might be. If the schema is always will to power-eternal return, we can understand how the category of repetition outside the grip of generality does not repeat the identical and the universal, but difference. It depends whether we get the point of the downright Artaudian "cruelty" of the idea, or not: *affective athleticism* (Artaud 1994). The turning-point is that of difference and the effect is the prolixity of the chaosmos, the production of life forms, actions and not mystique suspension.

The connection (*entrelacement*) of forces, whose seed is Will to Power, gives place to *a body*. More precisely, this relational connection of forces is the meaningful condition, the plot of *any body*. What is a body and what can a body do are questions about the same (*pseudo*) essence: "all reality is already quantity of force. There are nothing but quantities of force in mutual 'relations of tension'" (Deleuze 1983: 40), in the sense that if *all is* Will to Power, we must not forget that the seed of this whole is chaosmotic: totalizing in the sense of chaoticizing. It is the seed of an affirmative *autos*. So that when Deleuze writes, in harmony with Nietzsche, that the sense of a body is chance, "product of the forces of which it is composed", we have to think of the creativity inherent in the premises and precipitated into the outcome. In so far as it is a modulation present in a hierarchy of forces, a body is plural: "Being composed of a plurality of irreducible forces the body is a multiple phenomenon, its unity is that of a multiple phenomenon, a 'unity of domination'. In a body the superior or dominant forces are known as *active* and the inferior or dominated forces are known as *reactive*" (Deleuze 1983: 40). Quantity and quality are related and both contribute to define force in the singular relation of forces. The plurality that gives the hierarchy its life is a battle between "commanding" and "obeying". These qualities-quantities, the intensity of force, are in any case in relation to power, in the sense that they do not annihilate each other: commanding is not suppression but predominance. Active and reactive are the modalities expressing the forces in their relationship. Reactivity is the way in which the forces are more or less understood, introducing themselves as mechanism and/or finality. To understand forces as forces, however, their movement needs to be accepted in active modality. Both active and reactive, forces are the modular expression of force as Will to Power: both modes are the same. The activity is thought in the radically empirical sense as being plural from the start. To think the organism is to think of the specific dynamism that makes it up, to realize its form. From a merely anthropological point of view, its active-reactive relation is realized in the complex dynamic of self-consciousness to which Nietzsche draws attention, and which Deleuze refers to starting from the powers of the body before introducing his definition of consciousness, observing its moment of "modesty". Consciousness is such by virtue of forces in reactive modality: "It is not the master's consciousness but the slave's consciousness in relation to a master who is not himself conscious" (Deleuze 1983: 39).

The centrality of the life of the body is the affirmation of plural multiplicity as the creative source, in respect of which consciousness defines itself as a reactive retrospection, a relations of relations: the

Ego must think about its own re-sentiment or its own emotive resonances, for itself. The passage by Nietzsche from *Zarathustra, On the Despisers of the Body* (Nietzsche 2006: 22–24) is the reference. The thinking exercised by consciousness is therefore of *vital importance* and its being second with respect to the elusive richness of the activity of the Self, of which it is an approximate mouthpiece, does nothing to diminish its functionality, but it specifies it. It would be inappropriate to think of contesting Platonism against consciousness so as to imagine its denial in favour of the body. The overriding of Platonism and Cartesianism, with its priority given to the body rather than to some form of acephalous irrationalism, aims at the renewal of a new form of reason: in the name of incarnate reasoning and in the name of vital correspondence between thinking and affections, as an affect of the affections, or rather modulations of resonance in a becoming-body always open (Fadini 2015). The complex field of forces of the body and on all of the human body is seen as a place of *maximum experiment*: it is through the life of the body that it is possible to obtain a bio-blueprint of the *exceedance* and reconstruct a biography of complexity. In this sense, the body presents itself as an active horizon to which thinking reacts, which is why Deleuze writes: "What makes the body superior to all reactions, particularly that reaction of the ego that is called consciousness, is the activity of necessarily unconscious forces" (Deleuze 1983: 41–42), and: "the originality of Nietzsche's pluralism is found here. In his conception of the organism he does not limit himself to a plurality of constituent forces. What interests him is the diversity of active and reactive forces and the investigation of active forces themselves" (Deleuze 1983: 204).

Thinking, in this way, is seen as thinking *of* the body. Putting the emphasis on the differential means focusing attention on configuration and prevalence, and not on definitive exclusion. The immanent logic of this plural becoming-body indicates the basic grammar of a schizoid disjunctive synthesis in the name of *et-et* rather than *aut-aut* (Deleuze 1990). The composition between active and reactive forces characterizes – we might say 'colours' – the whole organism. Grasping at the active, as we said, is essential for understanding what force is and what the original really is. Activity is a plastic force, fully affirmative, aggressive, appropriative; it is *noble energy*. The reactive, on the contrary is that which can be grasped only in relation to the active, like consciousness with respect to the body (the resentment of a pain or a pleasure is, as we said before, a degree of reactive warning expressed by the consciousness, a fundamental function of the body, a diagonal way of achieving an aim of the body itself – the "great health").

The relationship between the forces, in Deleuze's Nietzschean pluralism, is a boundless original difference. Another key element to understand the question is given by the link between the quantity and quality of force. We have said that the forces are active or reactive; but force always has a quantity. The problem is to think the quantity in genealogical terms. Force, by its very nature, is always in relation, so that quantity will express itself not in abstract and absolute terms, assuming a scale of homogeneous measurement, but always and anyway as a difference of quantity with the quantity of another force: it is an approximate illusion to imagine two forces equal and have the opposite direction. Therefore, the quantity of force that we are dealing with here is the differential one, and so there is no need to try to reduce quantity to quality, it is enough to think of the concept of quantity on the right level of analysis. So, difference of quantity never leads to equality. Quality is difference of quantity in relation, on a level where there is no abstraction. The differential and the relational are the unavoidable substance of the relation inherent in the pluralism of Nietzschean empiricism, in contrast to the *metaphysical undifferential*.

Nietzsche's harsh criticism is against logical identity, mathematical equality, and physical equality: against the forms of the undifferentiated. It might be deduced that *we cannot count on the becoming* (in the sense of exhaustively and reassuringly enumerating stages as states): the point is that the becoming determines immeasurable chaining. The tendency to reduce differences of quantity corresponds to nihilism as an effort of negation and underestimation of the life in all its expressions. Compared to the conservation that evens in the undifferentiated, Nietzsche supports the differential force of profligacy. The idea of the Eternal Return of the Same is "synthetic" thought: "thought of the absolutely different [...] The eternal return is not the permanence of the same, the equilibrium state or the resting place of the identical. It is not the 'same' or the 'one' which comes back in the eternal return but return is itself the one which ought to belong to diversity and to that which differs" (Deleuze 1983: 46). And it is in this sense that one can speak of a terrible *must think* inscribed on the spirals of the eternal return of the same, since the form of a synthetic constructivism, so renewed in its depth, is the ultimate risk of thinking about the difference in its immanent affective mutation of forces. We have to grasp and establish the being of the becoming in those "cosmological" and "physical" terms which characterize the *chaosmos*. The becoming cannot become something, it has no beginning and end: nothing can be assumed about it. Following Deleuze's argument, thought of the pure becoming establishes the eternal return of the same.

"Pure becoming" assumes an ontology of time based on the "passing moment": to separate temporal ecstasy from its passing would bring about suspension in the undifferentiated and is a thought which might even be considered tendentious. It would be a distinction that measures by commeasuring, focused on the premise of an appearance-essence opposition. No distinction can be made between the instant and passage and we are therefore obliged not to believe any longer in a being separate from the becoming, but in a being *of* the becoming. This being is repetition: that all should return is the acme of "contemplation". It is not a question of linking together the present instants of an *Aion* which hinges on what is given, but of an *Aion* of the present as a passage. Contemplation and synthesis say the same thing: "The moment would not pass" if we should believe, like Bergson, that many juxtaposed stations of time do not make up real duration (Bergson 2001); or rather the condition of the passing of the moment is that it is not the sum of distinct, immobile presents. The contemplation-synthesis relation possessed by the passing moment ends up invalidating any logic of expectation which would in fact weaken and break up the wholeness and ontology of the pure becoming postulated as original. This, of course, is Zarathustra's vision and riddle: *the abyssal thought*. It is clear that the eternal return as such, on this level of pure experimentation, does not acknowledge that it supports a syntax of the eternal return itself as being 'of something', especially of the Same, assumed still to be in the form of recognition of a controllable differential. Deleuze is very clear on this point: the return not only does not belong to the being but it constitutes it; it is the return as affirmation of the becoming and of what passes in a way in which the "yes" is an opening and not an expectation. The "yes" changes the expectation into the opening of a new beginning; the return does not belong to the One, but makes *one* the affirmation of different. The affirmation of different is the alternative to negative distinction: the *individualized* is seen in its creative newness. "Identical" does not imply the being of that which returns as qualification of an object; or rather, this might be as so, if the *a priori* were the identity, and then one might think of an object to qualify, processed by the becoming. Instead, "Identical" connotes the return of the different. The principle by which the eternal return depends, its *sufficient reason*, is Will to Power.

Will to Power is *attributed* to a force but not as its predicate. It is absurd to propose any subject other than will, while imagining force as the subject of *will*. It is Will to Power that wills: there is no other subject with which it can be aligned or to which it can be delegated. The syntax of intimate attribution *will to power-force* must be interpreted quite differently. We said that force is essentially split in its size (or its excess) with which it is always in *relation*. The differential element between forces in relation is the mobile trait which at the same time constitutes its genetic element. *Split* implies that it is always in relation, *in-between*: *piece* without matrix, *among nubbles*, partial and integrable; *split* implies synthesis *in* and *of* multiplicity and quite clearly does not connote metaphysical distinction, nourished by the undifferential of the negative.

Will to Power as a sufficient principle and reason for the Eternal Return is a project of total freedom, which configures a chaosmos where the single project of nature-man would be called to overcome as care of becoming, since, in its specific, consciousness is a resentment of the activities of the forces and it is a necessary *regulator* of *affective* relations (and so it doesn't stand out as *The Law*). In this sense there could be a loss of anthropocentric prerogatives, wherever freedom is present, as we shall see, distributed-in it, and not attributed-to it; however, this probably loss of centrality does nothing more than empty of sense *a problem* of freedom seen as the "use and consumption", in view, on the contrary, to an ethical perspective of attention to the chaosmos with a much wider range and goes *from the world, one's own country, to one's neighbours, to oneself* (Deleuze 2011). In this way, the ethical rule (in place of the moral Law) is seen as projection of attention to a cycle which in reality is a *spiral*: a becoming-body in the name of synthetic, progressive constructivism.

Nothing further, then, by the surreptitious introduction of a *subjectum* with modern connotations in necessary response to a mystifying metaphysical question aiming to demolish and deconstruct this scene well built. An overcoming metaphysics exists in the serenity or joy (in Nietzschean terms) of a *hard-hitting* metaphysics in which the courage of the different is the full experimentation of the new. Not deconstructing metaphysics, but outlining a new image of thought.

Taken as a principle, the Will to Power unhinges the meaning of the transcendental, in view, however, of a form of superior empiricism (Palazzo 2013, Deleuze, *Fuori dai cardini del tempo. Lezioni su Kant*, edited by S. Palazzo, 2005). Like Nietzsche, Deleuze contests excess of the generality of principles in the classical sense. The Will to Power, on the contrary, "is a good principle, if it reconciles empiricism with principles, if it constitutes a superior empiricism", and this because "it is an essentially *plastic* principle that is no wider than what it conditions, that changes itself with the conditioned and determines itself in each case along with what it determines. The will to power is, indeed, never separable from particular determined forces, from their quantities, qualities and directions. It is never superior to the ways that it determines a relation between forces, it is always plastic and changing" (Deleuze 1983: 50).

This, then, is the reconfirmed track of Deleuzean transcendental empiricism. At this point we should underline what Deleuze considers to be the Nietzsche's "complex attitude" to Kant. While, on the one hand, Deleuze agrees with Nietzsche in attributing to Kant the discovery of the synthesis-concept, on the other he recuses Kant's principle as a basis for its functioning. To be more specific, the idea of total criticism developed by Nietzsche called for a revision of the notion of "condition" and therefore of "a priori". The criticism of the generality of principles relates directly to his "complex attitude" to Kant – a much more radical referent than the same dialectic. However one might see the arguments returned to and adopted, the principle of synthesis described by Nietzsche in Deleuze's interpretation is at the same time genesis and production. It is not a question of reversing, but to raise the issue of criticism, *ab origine*, on a different level of analysis (of high "resolution"), the level of immanence – how the principles *became* (by introducing the becoming into the same principle).

To maintain that Will to Power is inseparable from force, then, certainly does not mean that it is identical to it and reduced. Force *can*, Deleuze underlines, while will *wills*. This subtle statement involves the following dynamic: the *power* of force is in its ability to always establish a *relationship* of dominion; but this would be nihilistic if, for example, *dominated* force did not maintain its *vis* as intimate *will*. Precisely that which is the constitutive relation of the relation of dominion would not exist. Here we have plastic force where residuals of production are always produced. In symbolic and schematic terms, Deleuze summarizes the concept as dy/dx. This formula is easily explained in the light of we have already outlined in detail. If "d" stands for genealogical difference, differential characterised as the principle of Will to Power, and "x" and "y" are understood as representing forces, it emerges that Will to Power is to be taken as the genealogical element of force and forces simultaneously, preserving itself in the middle, as a substantive relation. Every living being is given a coefficient of Will to Power: the servant's will is not a will-negation, but its particular quality.

Now, interpretation and evaluation must take into account the "concrete physics" of forces, the whole battlefield, where it is all a question of "differences" (evaluation-creation). The interior battlefields is the hierarchy, where "free thinkers" and "free spirits" measure themselves against each other, typed reactive force – which proceeds to 'decompose', "by separating active force from what it can do" (Deleuze

1983: 64), by inoculation and contagion of the negative – and the active force, which behaves by *affirmation*. In this contrast are inscribed the characters of the two types of quality of force. It is interesting how slaves obtain victory: they do not triumph by summing each other in a total abstraction, but on the basis of the quality of the force that they are able to gain in specific terms, weakening active force and imposing their appreciative point of view. Theirs is always a subtraction: in other words, *even when a slave triumphs, he will never cease to be a slave*. So the problem of free spirits is to triumph in a *liberating* hierarchy and not, therefore, as slaves. So a free spirit can win only if his enemy wins too as free spirit. And above all, those who have "little force" are not slaves, but those are slaves who are in the condition of having their own force separated from that which is in their power. The free spirit is characterised, on the contrary, by the simple affirmation of his difference.

The Will to Power, recognized as such in the trait which modulates its dynamic differential, is seen as a fold: an epistemological fold. The ontology of the chaosmos is seen in the singular epistemological fold of a transcendental empiricism. And its *flap* results in a singular ethical perspective, so earning, in its eternal return, a *practical rule*.

Up to this point, we have discussed force and power without ever fully referring to the matter of the affections, which comes from Spinoza; the question of activity, in fact, is better understood if analyzed in the context of the affections. The determination of the relation between the forces is in the mark that one force leaves on the another: the relation is manifested as an affection. In fact, if Will to Power is the differential and genealogical element that determines the relation between forces, what it gives is evinced from the forces involved. Since it has special "good principle" characteristics, of a mesh not large enough to be larger than what it seizes to, Will to Power is a fold of relation in things/forces and it manifests itself "as a capacity for being affected" (Deleuze 1983: 62). This "capacity", of course, is not to be understood in terms of "abstract possibility". Here we have capacity for being affected, capacity that, as such, is present in every relation between forces. It might be imagined as a kind of bruise or scorch mark – the remains of production. It is at the same time a relation between forces as a moment in passing. The "double aspect" of the Will to Power is clearly this: from the standpoint of the genesis it determines the relation but, from the standpoint of its own manifestations, it is determined. The ambiguity that emerges induces us to think of the two sides of a fold and therefore it is *a fold*.

The capacity to be affected should not be confused with passivity. The fold makes us note that it is in the freedom of this principle to be split and therefore *capable* in its dynamism. Passivity in this sense stands for "*an affectivity,* a sensibility, a sensation" but we should again point out that this is the case in a superior empiricism. The fold of Will to Power, we might say, shows itself as "the primitive affective form" (Deleuze 1983: 62). In this sense, we realize that it is also considered to be a *pathos*, in its double meaning of experience-feel and experience-suffer at the same time. "Pathos is the most elementary fact from which a becoming arises" (Deleuze 1983: 63). And once again this duplicity is understood by Deleuze as the *differential* between the forces. Passivity as reception is internal to Will to Power; for this reason, the opposite or reverse of active is still re-active, as a way of experiencing/receiving the pathos of the forces. It is still a becoming which will produce itself in syntaxes of activity or re-activity. The power of being affected *between* the forces triggers processes of becoming sensitive.

How can a selection (hierarchy) between becoming-active or becoming-active of the forces be established? Assuming the eternal return as the practical rule, the forces are disentangled and the process, in one way or another, is selected: active-affirmative or reactive-nihilistic. The eternal return as a practical synthesis guides the will. To quote a fragment by Nietzsche of 1881: "If, in all that you will you begin by asking yourself: is it certain that I will to do it an infinite number of times? This should be your most solid center of gravity" (Deleuze 1983: 68). We have already explained the meaning of the eternal return: repetition. This is applied to the becoming and the becoming to that fold: to want the eternal return means wanting *as* the eternal return. It is an order that attests to how to will if the content of will is the eternal return. And as content, in its turn, the eternal return when applied to the becoming has that which we have called a differential fold. A Chinese-box construction shows us that content frees itself and we are faced with an extreme attempt at formalism: a radicalization of Kantian formalism with respect to whose dynamic no hypostasis holds. When the action supports its eternal return, it is fully creative: or rather *excess*, becoming-active. Extreme dissipation which, because of its total investment, affirms and gives place to the becoming-active. But note: a badly-supported eternal return is not a negation of the eternal return but only a falsification. A form of optimism is concealed in this new image of thought: an optimism beyond good and evil.

To quote again from *Zarathustra*: "Oh if only you would put aside all *half* willing and become as resolute in your sloth as in your deeds! Oh if only you understood my words: Go ahead and do whatever you will – but first be the kind of people who *can will*!" (Nietzsche 2006: 137, Deleuze 1983: 69). And Deleuze: "It is the *thought* of the eternal return that selects. It makes willing something whole. The thought of the eternal return eliminates from willing everything which falls outside the eternal return, it makes willing a creation, it brings about the equation 'willing = creating' " (Deleuze 1983: 69). It is true that a becoming-active might be produced; but that which produces the equation that frees is that which is redundant to freedom: the becoming-active of repetition is the only one that has a *being*, in the sense that we have used so far. In fact, where the becoming-active should assert itself as a being, where it is repeated in its synthesis, it is transmuted into becoming-active. And it *would know* how to will.

To summarize the argument so far:

1. The *chaosmos*, a synthesis of chaos and cosmos, *tyché* and *ananke*, is seen in what we have presented as the fold of Will to Power, sufficient reason for the eternal return of the same;
2. The eternal return of the same, by virtue of Will to Power understood as multiplicity, is the "good principle" of a new transcendental empiricism;
3. The freedom which emerges, on the crest of *chaosmos* and in its folds, appears to be absolute in the synthesis reproduced by the eternal return as a practical rule; but has quite a different appearance. In the first place, it is coessential to the fold of/in the *chaosmos*, and in this sense we can think of a freedom which is not attributed to a subject designated as if reduced to an extrinsic quality, but a Freedom distributed-in;
4. Distribution of freedom refers to the constitutive fact where the coessentiality between freedom and fold is in the dynamic and creative disproportion of the forces, therefore it is a *relational principle* given by/in the relation. If there is absoluteness (nothing is seen beyond this), it is in the *pathic* relation;
5. The anthropological specific is no longer to be understood on the level of a prerogative of moral freedom with the assumption of a subject of the modern kind, but in the quality of that being to be able to retroaction which, as care (discipline) of their affective forces (desire), might appear as care of the becoming in general;
6. Dynamic relationality as a principle, the difference intended as beginning by Deleuze as an interpreter of the Nietzschean philosophy of will, determines a substantial hetero-reference which, in the absence of the modern subject, finds its justification;
7. The body, or *a* body, as a force-field is, in its complexity, this freedom which frees, an excess (beyond all anthropomorphism, which is one an indication of a "reactive" parody). We call this concept of the body as "becoming-body", in that it has differential

and intensive traits, conceptually similar to the notion of "body without organs" (borrowed by Deleuze/Guattari from the work of Antonin Artaud, and used most frequently in *Capitalism and Schizophrenia*);

8. The last point, which we shall develop, is the effect of the practical "to be done": the need for education in the sense of training of the will for *free men*.

Echoing the militancy of *On the Genealogy of Morality*, a polemic work, Deleuze states that Will to Power has no need of strength, it is strength, on the contrary, which needs will. Against the enchainment of will to an object (and to a subject), like Nietzsche, Deleuze "announces" that the will makes you free in *excess* where it is "creation of new values" (it is to be remembered that Deleuze is basically referring back to the notorious "fabricated" work *Will to Power*, where this theme has the ethical meaning of the destruction and creation of new values). What might seem a monism of will is rather a distribution of multiplicity in redundancy. In this regard, the connection with a "pluralist typology" (Deleuze 1983: 86) can be explained. The 'type', compared to the *exemplum*, is not to be seen as being on the level of transcendent *hypostasis*, but rather 'chance', meeting – the scene is not one of a moralized planet, but of a Spinozistic ethical pluriverse.

The project of the critique is rooted in the dynamism of the fold of the Will to Power and is in appearance a design of an *unleashing* which, paradoxically, feeds on relation as an unalienable element. In the critique involved in the folds of the *chaosmos*, we find the paradox of a liberation which claims to be only a condition of a fully creative relation, expressed in joy. "Kant is the first philosopher who understood critique as having to be total and positive *as* critique. Total because 'nothing must escape it'; positive, affirmative, because it cannot restrict the power of knowing without releasing other previously neglected powers"; however, "he seems to have confused the positivity of critique with a humble recognition of the rights of the criticized [...] Kant saw critique as a force which should be brought to bear on all claims to knowledge and truth, but not on knowledge and truth themselves; a force which should be brought to bear on all claims to morality, but not on morality itself. Thus total critique turns into the politics of compromise: even before the battle the spheres of influence have already been shared out" (Deleuze 1983: 89).

The failure of critique so conceived is in a method incapable of fully maintaining the regime of immanence. With genealogy, an alternative dialectical logic is taken forward, so that legislation is creation.

Epistemology and ontology are clearly hit by an explosive charge activated by the device of Will to Power and the Eternal Return, so that
transcendental empiricism and plane of immanence live to the full the
same affirmation of freedom. A new thought (a new feeling) for a new
reality – and vice versa. The radical critique encourages the original
ethic-aesthetic of the becoming-body in the direction of a synthetic
constructivism.

Nietzschean perspectivism, which is deployed in the folds of its multiplicity, is the speculum by which the dynamisms of genealogy is
enlarged. The type (also the *critical type*) corresponds to perspectivism
and occupies it. Typology and topology are connected. The *critical type*
is the topical type of the eternal return: it wants its overcoming (it affirms
its difference). At this point, if it is still necessary, another misunderstanding needs to be cleared up. To tend towards affirmation in the same
way as towards freedom, to respond to freedom with freedom, is very
different from demanding freedom. This *moral* of the eternal return is
easily understood in its particular inclination for training, on which
Deleuze puts his emphasis. At point 8 above, we spoke of education as
one of the things "to be done". "Constrain to think" is culture, in the
sense of causing the active dinamism of freedom of "to be done": an
active training of the will – to power. To know how to will: to take risks,
create. "Not a method", writes Deleuze, "but a *paideia*, a formation, a
culture" (Deleuze 1983: 110), whose aim is the training of "free men",
in order to damage that of "the astonishing complicity of both victims
and perpetrators" (Deleuze 1983: 106), and again, to expose that
"monstrous vice […] which nature herself disavows and our tongues
refuse to name", of "voluntary servitude" (De La Boétie 1942: 4).

Training and health are the two ethical-aesthetic modalities pursued
by Deleuze/Nietzsche, like two tensors of liberation-affirmation in place
of the moral and religious binomial of education and salvation. In both
cases we have a *training* of the will (understood as complex multiplicity
of the body) whose commitment is in the transitivity of action in contrast
to reactions: to *act* reactions. The same emphasis on formation, in the
sense of "apprentissage" in relation to the "signs", is take up again in
M. *Proust et les signes* (Deleuze 2004), as testimony to the relevance of
the question from a purely immanent point of view.

Ontology, epistemology and ethics are intricate in the dynamism of
the eternal return: a new reality, new thought and new feeling. A new
feeling is the response to the pathic dynamism of the eternal return and
a new though cannot be separated from this feeling. A future of dynamic
freedom opens up these possibilities as expressions of the redundancy of
a difference in which all is risk and everything is utmost affirmative

experimentation. The subject's "to be done" involves a procedure and its necessity does not, on the basis of our premises, lie in an infinity that is always in act, but in the dynamic risk of a relational, pathic differential from which emerge unprecedented matters. The idea of overcoming expresses the movement of "returning" at more than one level – the being of repetition compared with the different. In Nietzsche's view, then, training and health are linked to the overcoming. Training and health, too, attest how much the fullness of the *body of the chaosmos* is always at stake as relationism, network, and a complex and irreducible combinatory interplay.

Culture and justice, differently from resentment (and from bad conscience) "constantly reveal the workings of a training activity". While resentment *breaks up* and produces expectations instead of inception, therefore hampering and restraint, the product of cultural activity is the free and active man: "the man who can promise" (Deleuze 1983: 134). Such a man is distinguished by being "supramoral", by *commutating* his reactive forces (also in the *cruelty* of pain), and his capacity to promise lives in him not being any longer guilty in any court of law: "It is he who speaks, he no longer has to *answer*". Note well, however, that in his overcoming he frees himself by the same process that has trained him: "culture is man's generic activity; but, since this activity is selective, it produces the individual as its final goal, where genericity is itself suppressed". The creation necessarily takes the place of knowledge, in a synthetic constructivism. Therefore, "the product of culture is not the man who obeys the law, but the sovereign and legislative individual who defines himself by power over himself, over destiny, over the law: the free, the light, the *irresponsible*" (Deleuze 1983: 137).

Affirmative fulfilment, repetition of difference, assumption acted out, tragic thought and philosophy of the will all point to the same path: the permutation of the will of nothing in the training of the Will to Power as an eternal return, or otherwise, but outside the language of Nietzsche, the disciplining of desire as care. The scenario of a synthesis of the multiple operated by the eternal return is the redundancy of relation where *absolute relativism* seems, in its condition of mystification, to be akin to an acclaimed form of reactivism. By the term *Nihil*, Deleuze means, in its Nietzschean sense, first and foremost "a value of nihil", a "depreciation of life" due to a fiction from which "worlds beyond the world" are born (Deleuze 1983: 147).

Thought – we can say at this point – is present as a complex "body". Knowledge is one of its *opportunities*, but not the only one. We said that the thought of the eternal return gives rise to a free response in the name of freedom; but where do you place the thought in order to think the

Will to Power and its eternal return? The bends of thought call for a *ratio cognoscendi* of the Will to Power quite distinct by a *ratio essendi*. In one case, the affirmative becomes dismissed from the Will to Power nourished by the negative; in the other, instead, the affirmative triumphs. One cannot know without working through the undifferential instrument of the negative. Just the same, one can and must think without it. In Deleuze, constructivism and training are constantly connected. New concepts are created by means of a free *to be done*; and thinking, on this sense, is a "throw of the dice". The main point, in which thought is permuted, is active destruction.

The affirmation of annihilation is cruelty, to refer again to Artaud, so it is the intensive that strikes the body without organs and not the *organs* which impose reactive paranoia to/in the body. The cruelty of affirmation is the great health of the body without organs: it is to look with the eyes of the sick at health, in order to find its poetic/poietic position in the world. When thought is pervaded by the *ratio essendi* of Will to Power, it changes the origin of its values. On this basis, one understands what Nietzsche is getting at and how he is opposed to every form of thought based on the powers of the negative, to every thought that moves with the negative element and to which the negation works as motor, power and quality.

Affirmation, in order to be such, implies destruction, otherwise we are witness to a sinister attempt at justification of the real (or of *infinity in act*), which rests on premises we have attempted to remove. In this regard, a description of ass's character well illustrates the argument. The ass (or the camel) *affirms by accetance* without taking action. His is not a *Ja sagen*, but the A-I/A-I of braying. This acoustic image, so disrespectful, pronounces a yes incapable of saying no: "acquiescing in the real as it is, taking reality as it is upon oneself [...] The idea of the real in itself is an ass's idea. The ass feels the weight of the burdens that it has been loaded with, that it has taken up, as the positivity of the real. What happens is this: the spirit of gravity is the spirit of the negative, the combined spirit of gravity is the spirit of the negative, the combined spirit of nihilism and reactive forces" (Deleuze 1983: 181) Yes cannot rank as a function of being or of what it is: a function of the being present in the cosmos, under the threat of chaos. This Yes is also the absolution of the indifferential. The yes of adequacy is the acceptance of a real assumption as something already given and indisputable, revealed.

On the contrary: *"To affirm is not to take responsibility for, to take on the burden of what is, but to release, to set free what lives. To affirm is to unburden: not to load life with the weight of higher values, but to create new values which are those of life, which make life light and* active. There is creation, properly speaking, only insofar as we make use of excess in order to invent new forms of life" (Deleuze 1983: 185). The Yes of the *theatrum philosophicum* of the eternal return, *the theatre of cruelty*, is the index expressing of Nietzschean pluralism, in which radical empiricism and ethos dovetail in the (acted out) assumption of a superior experimentation.

To quote a famous statement from *Etichs*, Deleuze writes: "Spinoza [...] said that we do not even know what a body *can do,* we talk about consciousness and spirit and chatter on about it all, but we do not know what a body is capable of, what forces belong to it or what they are preparing for" (Deleuze 1983: 39), and its capacity, as we have seen, is in its power/potential to be affects. From the great Spinoza-Nietzsche identity, made possible by the fusion of the pure ontology of the Dutch philosopher and the device of the eternal return of the same as practical Nietzschean philosophy, Deleuze manages to establish a new verticality of the body (plural postures of the becoming-body), with the intention of freeing it from the dominion not characterized by negative subtraction but by positive affirmation, so that from the forces we pass to the affections, from these to desire and finally to desiring-machines, by means of multiple hetero-references conjunction vectors.

The ethical plane of immanence introduced by Spinoza allows the traditional metaphysical question about essence, "What is it?" to be transposed into the question about a differential quantity, "What can it do?" The question, therefore is to ask ourselves about the "modes of existence" and the question immediately becomes plural: "When, a long time after Spinoza, was Nietzsche to launch the concept of 'will to power', that is to say, *but not only,* this", and Deleuze intervenes, clearing up all (recurrent) misunderstanding, which propels the dynamic "Modal" and "quantitative" of power into a collapse of *potency* (as effective potential) and power: "Will to power means defining things, men and animals in relation to the effective potential they might have. This brings us constantly back to the same question: What can a body do? (Deleuze 2010). Power, in fact, is presented as an "affection of desire" in the complex argument of *Anti-Oedipus* (Deleuze/Guattari 2000), and therefore, shall we say, a specific case of the forms taken by a becoming-body.

On the shifting sands of the affections, it has no meaning to postulate a *proprium* of human nature in a predetermined order of ontic eminences, and it is for this reason, in Deleuze's opinion, that Spinoza seems to have no interest in discussions of a concept of freedom as belonging to human nature. The question is a different one: "What does it mean, *becoming free,* once it is said that we are not? We are not born free, we are not born reasonable. We are completely at the mercy of encounters, that is: we are completely at the mercy of decompositions […] the authors who think that we are free by nature are the ones who make of nature a certain idea. […] If you conceive yourself as a collection of relations, and not at all as a substance, the proposition 'I am free', is plainly deprived of sense. It is not at all that I am for the opposite: it makes non sense, freedom or not freedom. On the other hand, perhaps the question has a sense: How to *become* free?" (Deleuze 2010: 128).

From Deleuze's viewpoint, we can say that thinking freedom *in its essence* starting from nothing (*Nihil*) is to misunderstand the concept and limit its range (and to betray the strength by re-proposing it in the guise of an *eminent* power); conversely, if we pose the question in terms of the affective forces, its assumes the full sense of becoming-free (making-free) as affirmative construction. It is, then, a question of creating optimal relations. In this case, freedom is not the opposite of *connection* (the interdependence of the existing human mode); it is rather the opposite of "*sad*" – where 1) we are always in relation; 2) sadness is a *relation* suffered as *separation*.

So the becoming-free is always in the differential fold (of chaosmos), as a partition and remodeling of belongings *in progress*. The *path* of formation (training) of/in the becoming-body, as building up and breaking down individuality/singularity, it is not such unless it contemplates risks and not such, above all, unless it is proposed as a start.

What can a body do? is a question about growth and emotional training – of conjugation of/in freedom: "*apprentissage*" in the name of "signs" – and not of "symbols", where the notion of "symbol" refers to metaphysical Signifiers.

"Spinoza saw drives, motivations, emotions, and feelings – an ensemble Spinoza called affects – as a central aspect of humanity. Joy and sorrow were two prominent concepts in his attempt to comprehend human beings and suggest ways in which their lives could be lived better", writes the neurobiologist Damasio (Damasio 2003: 8), finding in the overall inspiration of the Dutch philosopher a way of reflecting useful for recounting his research on the relation between emotions, feelings and the brain, maintaining that the feelings are precious "biological sentinels" specializing in the aim to conserve, but also improving, life. The question "What can a body do?" described in terms of self-discipline, expresses itself as care for the feelings. The "what it feels like" is the unavoidable place of a post-subjectivity open for *redundant* constructive hetero-references.

Transcendental empiricism, so stigmatized by Deleuze in his particular synthesis of Spinozian and Nietzschean thinking, resulting in the exemplary categorization of the plane of immanence, or plane of consistency, in the work with Felix Guattari, *What is Philosophy?* (Deleuze/Guattari 1994), brings back into thinking the condition of the *thinkability* of the affections and of relational hetero-reference as a prerequisite of any form of identity, in the name of a purely affirmative freedom. This model seems to be functional, then, to a reformulation of the fundamental anthropological question in the sense of a renewed synthetic posthuman constructivism which, given substantial mutation, contemplates the specific human case as a sign of care of a becoming-free at plural, starting from a becoming-body, so that this occasion for an interdisciplinary rethink of the anthropological subject produces further occasions for communal emancipation against any forms of enslavement and subjugation.

Bibliography

Artaud, A. 1994: *The Theatre and its Double*, trans. M. C. Richards. New York: Grove Press.

Bergson, H. 2001: , trans. F. L. Pogson. Mineola (New York): Dover Pubblications.

Damasio, A. 2003: *Looking for Spinoza. Joy, Sorrow, and the Feeling Brain*. London: Heinemann.

De La Boétie, E. 1942: *Discourse on Voluntary Servitude*, trans. H. Kurz. New York: Columbia University Press.

Deleuze, G., 1969: *Spinoza et le problème de l'expression*. Paris: Edition de Minuit.

Deleuze, G. 1983: *Nietzsche and Philosophy*, trans. H. Tomlinson. New York: Columbia University Press.

Deleuze, G., 1990: *The Logic of Sense*, trans. M. Lester. New York: Columbia University Press.

Deleuze, G. 1991: *Empiricism and Subjectivity. An Essay on Hume's Theory of Human Nature*, trans. C. V. Boundas. New York: Columbia University Press.

Deleuze, G. 1994: *Difference and Repetition*, trans. P. Patton. New York: Columbia University Press.

Deleuze, G. 1995: *The Exhausted*, trans. A. Uhlmann. Madison: University of Wisconsin Press.

Deleuze, G. 2003: *Spinoza. Philosophie pratique*. Paris: Les Editions de Minuit.

Deleuze, G. 2004: *Proust and Signs*, trans. R. Howard. Minneapolis: University of Minnesota Press.

Deleuze, G., 2004: *Fuori dai cardini del tempo. Lezioni su Kant*, trans. S. Palazzo, Milano, Mimesis (see also *La voix de Gilles*).

Deleuze, G. 2010: *Cosa può un corpo?*, trans. A. Pardi, Verona, Ombre Corte (see also *La voix de Gilles*).

Deleuze, G. 2011: *Gilles Deleuze From A to Z* (with C. Parnet), trans. C. G. Stival. Cambridge: MIT Press (DVD).

112 ROSELLA CORDA

Deleuze, G., Guattari, F. 1987: *A Thousand Plateaus. Capitalism and Schizophrenia*, trans. B. Massumi, Minneapolis: University of Minnesota Press.

Deleuze, G., Guattari, F. 1994: *What Is Philosophy?*, trans. H. Tomlinson and G. Burchell. New York: Columbia University Press.

Deleuze, G., Guattari, F. 2000: *Anti-Oedipus. Capitalism and Schizophrenia*, trans. R. Hurley *et al*. Minneapolis: University of Minnesota Press.

Deleuze, G., Guattari, F. 2003: *Kafka: Toward a Minor Literature*, trans. D. Polan. Minneapolis: University of Minnesota Press.

Fadini, U. 1993: L'identità Spinoza-Nietzsche. Movimenti filosofici in Deleuze. *Fenomenologia e società*.

Fadini, U. 2015: *Divenire-corpo. Soggetti, ecologie, micropolitiche*. Verona: Ombre Corte.

Heidegger, M. 1979: *Nietzsche I. The Will to Power as Art*, trans. D. F. Krell. New York: Harper & Row.

Heidegger, M. 1984: *Nietzsche II. The Eternal Recurrence of the Same*, trans. D. F. Krell. New York: Harper & Row.

Marchesini, R. 2002: *Post-human. Verso nuovi modelli di esistenza*. Torino: Bollati Boringhieri.

Masullo, P. A. 2008: *L'umano in transito. Saggio di antropologia filosofica*. Bari: Edizioni di Pagina.

Nietzsche, F. 1994: *The Birth of Tragedy out of the Spirit of Music*, trans. S. Whiteside. London/New York: Penguin Books.

Nietzsche, F. 1998: *On the Genealogy of Morality*, trans. M. Clark and A. Swensen. Indianapolis: Hackett Publishing Company.

Nietzsche, F. 2006: *Thus Spoke Zarathustra. A Book for All and None*, trans. A. Del Caro. Cambridge/New York: Cambridge University Press.

Nietzsche, F. 2008: *Twilight of the Idols or How to Philosophize with a Hammer,* trans. D. Large. Oxford: Oxford University Press.

Palazzo, S. 2013: *Trascendentale e temporalità. Gilles Deleuze e l'eredità kantiana*. Pisa: ETS.

Scheler, M. 1926: Man and History. In *Philosophical Perspectives*, trans. O. Haac. Boston: Beacon, 1958, 65–93.

Scheler, M. 2009: *The Human Place in the Cosmos*, trans. M. S. Frings. Evanston: Northwestern University Press.

Spinoza, B. 1996: *The Ethics*, trans. E. Curley. London/New York: Penguin Books.

Zaoui, P. 1995, La grande identité Nietzsche-Spinoza. Quelle identité? *Philosophie* 47, 64–84.

CHAPTER

8

The Pathosophie[1] of the Posthuman

PAOLO AUGUSTO MASULLO

The posthuman is the irreducibile 'fact' deriving from the process of changes in cognitive states that, during the twentieth century, triggered a 'revolution' in the possible paradigms that can be used, among other things, for a new and necessary definition of the image of man and human identity. Because of these changes, this 'fact', which the term posthuman primarily designates, derives from the dissolution of the overall modern anthropocentric humanistic paradigm and from the emergence of an anthropodecentric paradigm that is called posthuman.

The humanistic paradigm was already being systematically rethought, in fact, at the beginning of the twentieth century with the birth of philosophical anthropology as an independent discipline; this came about formally in 1928 with the publication of Max Scheler's *Die Stellung des Menschen im Kosmos* (Scheler 2009) and his proposal for a methodological integration of the general theory of the concept of the human and our specific knowledge of man. Max Scheler was working on the reformulation, in a new humanistic key, of the concept of the humanity of man and his philosophic possibility by means of the construction of a paradigm that would stand up in the light of science, all that was properly positive-naturalistic (chemistry, physics, etc.) and all that was "historical-natural" (biology, psychology, etc.), significantly introducing them, in his investigation of the issue, as being disciplines appropriate for the essential definition of man but, at the same time, giving them associations beyond such a definition by the precise identification of the "specialty" of the human in man which, compared to every other living being, was regarded, in terms of its irreducible difference, as being "supernatural" and cosmic, of the spirit (*Geist*). In his main work, *Der Mensch* (Gehlen 1988), Scheler's disciple Arnold Gehlen rejected Scheler's metaphysical approach and identified the human specialty in a defective human condition, man as a "would-be being", *Mängelwesen*, from the prerequisitively biological-natural point of view, and saw the possibility of man's "salvation" in the anthropocentric structure of a "second nature", that is culture, actually describing it as a discontinuous model with a nature-culture dichotomy. This specialty, however, from the evolutionary point of view, turned out to be nothing less than the "construction of a particular positioning in the world" so that "it is not possible to consider the epistemic anthropocentric prospect as being objective, universal, and subsumptive; it is, however, biased, specialized and unbalanced" (Marchesini 2014: 47; see also 2002). If it is the evolutionary process that governs the transformative flux of life and the living being, it seems evident that also "the cognitive function is a product of adaptive specialization, and for this reason [...] it is not better than the cognitive modes of other species", because it is only one of the possible modes of adaptation inevitably intended to produce "interpretative alterations", or partiality and reconfigurations of context". This means that "anthropocentric epistemy", as one of the many functions of the species-specific cognitive worlds, is not better than that of other species and is not objective, not neutral and [...] cannot be used as a unit of measurement to evaluate heterospecific epistemics" (Marchesini 2014: 48).

The posthuman therefore seems to be a child of the epistemological outcomes of Darwinian evolutionism which brings down so many of the pillars of western humanistic thought.

Philosophical anthropology, therefore, in its brief life of a few decades, is not able to explain the radical transformations of epistemic context first introduced by biology and by its amazing development as a 'historical' rather than a 'non-naturalistic' discipline, and then by the ever-increasing development of the same biological knowledge empowered by technological knowledge and by their progressive merging and dialogue.

As a result, the humanistic paradigm, even as soon as the early 1950s, was already deprived of its basic epistemological categories, quite apart from those which are properly philosophical. During the everyday practices of the acquisition of knowledge, old dichotomies which were no longer sustainable gradually fell out of use: for example, the dichotomies nature/culture, human/animal, biological/technological, natural/artificial, etc., which even suggest a rethinking of the most traditional of the basic disjunctive dichotomies of the humanistic-naturalistic tradition (that is, radically "non-natural"): that oppositive disjunction, never positively demonstrated as such, which is ascribed to Aristotle, *Bios* and *Zoé*. We are seeing the opposite, a progressive conceptual return to the "connective" type, to be considered as a positive methodology which is gradually changing the cognitive epistemic status of the human being;

this reconnection is aimed at the recognition of a *continuum* which is gradualistic, adaptive, multi-level and provisional (Masullo 2008, Braidotti 2013) which will definitively release the old idea of unitary human identity from specious dichotomous and disjunctive concepts. Furthermore, all ideas of a solid and stable definition of the human and the identity of man seem to be exposed to the progressive and inexorable crumbling of a building constructed on the basis of the perhaps outdated belief according to which it is fully demonstrated that life, because of its biological processes, is irrevocably destined to an inevitable historically-demonstrated transformation rather than a rigid permanence naturalistically based on laws which are more or less eternal (Mayr 1982, 2004). Basic theoretical elements about the deposition of the traditional categorization of the humanistic paradigm, at the ideal theoretical level, in principle and sequentially, the failure of that attempt at rationalization of the world based on the concept of a solid monolithic form of theoretical reasoning (*mathesis universalis*) separable in all its parts from the living body, that which gives man a stable identity, progressively eliminating all its pre-individual constitution, other than its consciousness, which is founded on the emotions, which have always been thought of as an "impure" natural residual (Marchesini 2002), that is, on that preindividually emotional makeup (*patica*) that is understood as belonging to the original and "inevitable" horizon of the process of life.

In relation to the constitutive and constituent horizon of identity, the ideas of Gilbert Simondon are of great importance. He points out, among other things, that "the intimacy of the individual [...] should not be sought at the level of pure organic consciousness or unconsciousness, as much as at the level of the affective-emotive subconscious [...] This relational stratum is the centre of individuality." (Simondon 2005: 242–243). Here, in fact, we are looking, in terms of humanistic modernity, at the definitive separation of mind and body, *logos* and *pathos*, a separation which is nicely turned upside-down and then uprighted in the appropriate hierarchical order only in the approach adopted by Nietzsche in the nineteenth century. Nietzsche's philosophy makes the living body central again in the only possible form, *Pathos*. As a production system, in fact, the living body, among the other ways in which it expresses itself, "realizes" the "function" of reasoning; the centralizing of the living human body, and its essential affective character, by no means implies the assumption of an anthropocentric perspective. It does imply, however, in terms of the changes still occurring today, the basic "neutral" existence – for the living – of a constitutive "patho-centric" position.

In Nietzsche's brief essay of 1873, *Über Wahrheit und Lüge im außermoralischen Sinne* (edited in 1895), we read: "But if we could communicate with a midge we would hear that it too floats through the air with the very same pathos, feeling that it too contains within itself the flying centre of this world" (Nietzsche 1873: 141). Pathos-centrism means that it is not man who is cental, but his *pathos*, which is the *pathos* of every living individual which has its centre in the *pathic*. So that pathos-centrality, both individually and comprehensively, is the form of life itself.

The "patho-centric" living individual dimension, in its turn, redefines "that which can be renamed psychic individuality" and research into the living human, instead of being logically rejected, "should concentrate on the affections and the emotions" (Simondon 2005: 243). Affectivity and emotivity are characteristics not only of man but of every living being. "The quantum regime of affectivity and emotivity" should be seen as being "at the centre of the individual", that is in accordance with research "into the structure and the genesis of all species and organisms: no living being would seem to lacking in affectivity-emotivity, which is quantum in complex beings like man just as it is in beings of poor organization" (2005: 243). It is from reflections such as these that we realize that the anthropocentric myth has now collapsed, starting from the very image of Vitruvian Man based on the logical-rational idea of man as the "centre" and "measure of all things".

Anthropocentrism, therefore, is not an expression of *hybris*, of arrogance, in the tradition of Promethian mythology, but an illusion, a need for stability and reassurance which, however resistant it may be in its cold rationality, is irrevocably non-sustainable in the dynamic process of the evolutionary continuum. In every living being, whether simple or complex, "there is evidence of affectivity-emotivity which act as the basis for inter-subjective communication" (2005: 243).

The "patho-centric" hypothesis, even when modified by the Plessnerian hypothesis which recognizes a specific human character in the concept of *eccentricity* (Plessner 1981) is clear evidence of the radical crisis of the modern Subject; at the height of its "anthropo-logo-centric" creation, it is developing rapidly and taking on a new dimension in the idea of a multicentric subjectivity which can be represented as a multicentric subjectivity based primarily on the affective-emotive. It is also the result of a staggering area of research in the new concept of consciousness which can no longer be seen simply as an expression of a monolithic I, but only partly certifiable as the manifestation of a series of events to be classified in a sequence of degrees and states differing and varying in mode and intensity which are more or less regularly fuelled from outside by experience of alterations and, from inside, by something obscure and incomprehensible, living/emotional. This, in its turn, is nothing more than a "background movement" (consciousness in general or, rather, the non-conscious) which, moving from bottom to top, towards the surface towards the exterior to become what is literally a phenomenon, fuels the border/space, uncertain and multiform, of the phenomenal conscious act and the cognitive phenomenon, expressed in all its various degrees. In the course of this process of emancipation of presumptuous and spurious anthropocentric centrality, this is a transition from the vacuum, the intangible and hypostatically metaphysical "formal Subject", a refuge protected from the world and a purely illusory centre, to a multicentric subjectivity, "nomad" in the sense that it is constantly on the move. In this epoch-making transition, then, we hace an essential variation of the concentrative and regular intensivity of the terms *logos*, subject, Ego, "reason", consciousness, which has gradually taken on the identity of a consequent "change of density": while modernity, with its origins in the idea of man being the centre of all things, is built around the Subject (*psyche*, soul, reason, consciousness, mind, io) as an increasingly dense coagulation of human identity, tending towards a typically humanistic separation from the living world in a anthropologo-centric position by means of which man's identity is a "must-be" obligation according to the model of a presumably absolute rational principle, with the arrival of the "crisis of the modern", the subject, having become a mere "metaphysical hypostasis" , has gradually "diluted" or "dilated" to the point where it has assumed a "multicentric" character or, if one prefers, the "peripherical" character of the "nomad subject" or of *"multiplex* singularity". The change of identity of the Id, especially because of the rarefaction of the centric subject, does not mean we should eliminate subjectivity, but that we should move to an idea of its multidirectional patho-centric expansion: less "subject-(mono)centric" and more widespread peripherical or multicentric subjectivity. With its expansion, the subject, traditionally thought of as the kernel or original nucleus, *Ich-Kern* (Pfänder 1911), now thins out. As it acquires new operative terrain and externalizes itself by the expansion brought about by the bio-techno-info-medial explosion, it becomes less dense. Its rarefaction is dilution of the centre and also a process of increasing exteriorization, an *acting out*: a coming-out that might also run the risk of becoming an "all-outside" or an "only-outside", with resulting exhaustion of all possible inner being. The process is a double movement of "away-from", both horizontal and vertical: a moving away from the centre, "Id-nucleus" (*Ich-Kern*), and from the bottom (*hypokeimenon, sub-jectum*) as a simultaneous movement away from the central-Id and the bottom-essence. It is in this process of "dilution", a phenomenon which is increasingly evident, that the "fact" of the posthuman lies.

This anthropological reconfiguration means that we are progressively going beyond the traditional borders of the above and the below, inside and outside. A structuring of stratified and multiple identity is taking shape which tends to include in positive life, also, for example, the experience of estrangement, of distancing *from the self*, of distancing *of the self*. Hence, it is rarefaction by horizontal dilution, starting from a centre, and a vertical movement away from the bottom to the surface. From dentitary centre, subjectivity has acquired a scattered and dispersive identity; from the firm ground of the Id, it has become a completely exteriorized and unidentified landscape. In conclusion, it is transformed and is configured in *nomad* subjectivity (Deleuze/Guattari 2000 and 2005, Braidotti 1994).

In this new picture, typical of the posthuman landscape, identity, then, becomes an individual option chosen and self-realized by innumerable available tools which permit discrete and variable self-construction, flexible and multiple.

The posthuman, therefore, means "the crumbling away of the metaphysical barrier [...] that separated the ego from social and natural reality" and therefore "the individual (*multiplex*) [...] is spilling into the world of immanence. The refuge of consciousness [...] appears but is also dragged out of the 'Heraclitean' river of incessant transformation" (Bodei 2004: 251). The idea of human identity having as its basis a new epistemy is changing, together with its openness to new, multiple and imaginative modes of existence, structuring a desired reconfiguration which has a new permanent possible development. This new dynamic, typical of the posthuman, defers "to a widespread human sample that finds it pleasant to live with a multiple and malleable ego [...] that wishes to experience many "parallel lives" [...] visiting multiple "vital worlds" or fitting into different spheres of belonging" (2004: 261).

In the changing identity of the human being as announced by the posthuman, it is possible to represent a new form of the ego which it would be better to call, in terms of subjectivity, simply as "general self-referentiality" for reasons of affection and which might be defined as the *modular me* in which the multiplicity of identities, having as their basis a constant condition of virtuality, manage to create in "almost-real" time a complex system of experimentable "singularities" in a wide field of space/time; a multiplicity which is always available because, for example, it is always at hand though the development of *networks*, of virtual reality, of the medial society, and is ready for the possible explosion, relative and relational, of the global structure capable of interlocutively including every self-alteration of living beings and the environment.

The posthuman is therefore enabling us to create, as a descriptive category, the position that man has found himself occupying following certain historically-significant turning-points in the process of consciousness and development, modeled on the Western tradition of thought, that have radically modified ontology, transforming it into "historical ontology" or an historical dimension of the living being with special reference to the man-entity, which is to be considered mainly as a (philosophical) anthropology in development. The human being, it is argued, can be investigated for any purpose and in accordance with any epistemy, only by means of an historical-evolutionary model while at the same time, reformulating in a continual process of self-improvement the idea of the possible human.

In particular, and from the point of view that is proposed here, as we investigate the by-now visible horizon of the posthuman, it appears to be worthy of attention to take up again the question of the affections (*the pathic*) to be understood from the methodological angle, and from that of the present writer, as the interpretive key to the human being in general and, taken here to be the object of the investigation, as the differential element in the new phase characterizing the posthuman.

The argument put forward here takes as its starting point the great anthropology lessons with a patho-centric focus for which, on the one hand, we have Baruch Spinoza's "Desire in given affection of itself" (Spinoza 2002: 311), and on the other Friedrich Nietzsche's reason is "a state of relations between different passions and desires" (Nietzsche 2006: 236); these are the first working theses in the history of humanistic modernism. In accepting such premises, and especially in relation to Nietzsche, we need to ask what was "the state of relation between (human) passion and desire" that produced an idea of reason, in the modern sense of "humanistic turning-point", used merely to refer to its calculating power, as a formal part of discourse on the "arithmocratic" model, in the unconfessed wish to make reason the "unique passion". We need to ask what those relations were, however "sick" they might have been, when we consider the outcomes of that model of rationalization that was used in the undertakings of modernity in the devastating tragedy of the two world wars. This is a question that, together with all its horror, should still be on the lips of those believers in a logo-anthropocentric and disjunctive humanistic model based on an idea of reason that engages only with the "affection" *Sollen*, that is moral obligation. This obligation, as last affection, appeared in the process of evolution and is perhaps the least "natural-vital" compared with the five Weizsäckerian *pathe*; though necessary to human coexistence, we so often do not understand what it is and, above all, to *whom* it might refer in the modern age if not blindly to the wielding of power of the few or, in the best of cases, to the meaningless punishment of ourselves.

Spinoza and Nietzsche, therefore, have given us powerful arguments against any idea of the purity of anything that might be attributed to man as an essence or a faculty like the logical-rational. At the same time, their respective ideas allow us to move away from the basic assumption that human life, with all its characteristics, can *tout court* be dynamically considered, interpreted and studied, perhaps in order to understand it, on the basis of the "affections", whose historical explanation in the becoming changes according to temporal orders that are more or less stable and according to moments of "rupture" and transformation. We are therefore convinced that research into the difference between the human and the posthuman should certainly move away from the affec-tive-emotive level (*the pathic*) and that it is able, though analysis, genealogies and perspectives of transformative identities, to understand the dynamically open and historically variable meaning of the possible definitions of human and posthuman identity. "The affective-emotive is a movement from indeterminate nature to the *hic et nunc* of present-day existence: it corresponds to that reality by which the indetermine subject moves to the present." (Simondon 2005: 247).

Therefore, the crisis of the human, or rather, of humanistic (rational) thought/*logos* the total colonizer of thought/affection when it is not its suppressor, marks the breakup of a historical order, that is a certain his-torical configuration of human life and identity, a breakup that occurs through culture, and, as we have said, it introduces another: the 'fact' of the posthuman, the critical framework which the model of thought/*logos* constructed in the modern age has begun to dissolve, giving way to a new form of expression of affection/life which is even more difficult to define but which might belong to the general category of certain possibly think-able forms which are totally 'other' and which can be investigated by using the image and meanings of thought/affection.

The expression "thought/affection", which belong to the above-mentioned categories of the *pathic* as described in the explanatory note to the title of this essay, *The Pathosophie of the Posthuman*, is meant the entire emotional repertoire of life, from the level of the structures and processes of its basic biological materials – one might say from the "primordial emotions" (Denton 2005) to the most complex affective expressions of the emotions and conscious feelings, in the web of a continuum that is a general expression of the living being and, in particular, the forms of expression of the living human being which themselves constitute its definition.

Firstly, in the time of the posthuman, the typical question of the modern age, "What is man"? seems to be undergoing a crisis. The next and innovatively transformed twentieth century question, "Who is man?", as a question about the identity of whoever says "I" and which is an early form of significant anthropological decentralization, is now accompanied by, and in some way replaced by the powerful new question, pregnant with meaning, which probes into the process of change: "What is man becoming?" In other words: "What will he who says 'I' become?" Which, from this moment on, is to ask how transformations, which have speeded up today as never before, might be able to define the prospects of that specific living being that we have been, that we are today, and that we might be tomorrow, among all the many products of the 'womb' of life, given that, in the anthropodectralisation process, ready to dialogue with animal otherness and, even more surprisingly, ready to fully recognize technological otherness, without prejudice to our own patho-centricity, which we have in common with every order and degree of living being.

Not only, then, do we have to call the past into question, we also have to plan a future with its 'maybe' and 'how'. The 'maybe' includes the possibility, in transformation, of remaining human, even if 'post-'; the 'how' questions *how* we are becoming and can become, between the poles of what we are no longer, merely human, and what we are becoming, posthuman. So man, whether as a single individual or a species-specific genus, is learning to look at himself no longer as a fact, but as a to-do, as a *work in progress*. The human being, therefore, must be seen as the expression of a transitive, as well as transitory, animal condition in constant transformation because of his hybrid constitution, which today is either completely ceasing to be, or at least, through bio-technoscience, modifying its species-specific identity.

Every single production of an object which is added to the available affective-symbolic order, modifies our relational perception of/with the world and our effective range of performance. The more bio-technoscience is able to produce high-performance objects in its dialogue with our pathocentric subjectivity, the more "thought/affection" is modified, so multiplying our identity-perceptions through the constant reconfiguration of the relations between the *pathei*.

The variations in the affections, through the *pathei*, described by the neurophysicist Viktor von Weizsäcker, which have inspired the two themes of this book as well as the title of this essay, have a marked profound changes in the passage from a disjunctive anthropocentric model to a non-disjunctive, multicentric anthropology as an indicator of the passage from the old model of the human to the new model of the posthuman.

If we admit, in accordance with the point of view taken in this essay, that the living human identity, in its relation *to* the world, dynamically "self-constitutes" its form of development and transformation across the range of the affections/emotions, the increasingly rapid change in the dialogical reference framework compared with a world/environment reconfigured by means of animal, and not only human, otherness, and now, especially, by means of machine otherness as the main interlocutionary referents, it seems evident that we need to rethink the ways by which human identity and subjectivity are being constructed and reconstructed.

Technological and bio-technological devices are increasingly able to govern the processes of desire and the affections which are the fundamental expression of the vital and the living. The transformed interlocation with non-human, animal and machine otherness is increasingly redefining our affective fields and changing the modulation, intensity and typology of our desires. Obligation, as an unavoidable necessity imposed by the 'natural' order (aging, falling sick or dying), will (as the practice of active desire), ability (as the expression of the possibility of action), and even moral obligation (as the only more specifically human affection compared with living beings in general) within the framework of radical change of the environment – which has become a techno-environment in which the living being man behaves – change profoundly, varying the dimensions and the relationships of reciprocal relation between the *pathei* in the sphere of the affective/emotive order. Technologies, and above all bio-technologies, greatly transform the dimension and relationship between the affective/emotive states of living human subjectivity. One case of such changes may be seen, for example, in the new techincal modalities of subjective medial experience ("post-medial") that can be experienced thanks to the interaction of different technological devices: this is the experience of the so-called *first personal shot*, a kind of "hypersubjective" video shot used in a great many videogames, films and image productions which show "the presence of an incorporated, dynamic and relational expression in the eyes; an intimate synergy of this body glance and a camera lens [...] in which the subject of the action of the experience constitutes itself dynamically and interactively" (Eugeni 2015: 61). Therefore changing his perception of himself and multiplying the modes of his experience, changing the affective/emotive orders of doing, of ability and being able, and so on.

The multicentrism of subjectivity, or rather, and epistemologically speaking, its "a-centrism" caused by loss or multiplication tending to the infinite, of a logical/identity centre, which is typical of the posthuman condition, derives from the consideration – again, typical of the cognitive sciences – that redefines subjectivity as being a "necessity" on the basis of the chaotic order of perceptions, actions, emotions, all representations into which the individual finds himself 'thrown'. We are life that evolves because the "original subjectivity" of life, as a patho-centrism of every single living individual, is the specific character of being a "form of life" (Masullo 2014). It is a power able, though not necessarily, to attain and arrive at a significant subjectivity by gradually constructing and self-constructing to the point of being a self-aware and reflexive subjectivity. The degree of this self-awareness and reflexivity, when it reaches the human level, is called a 'subject' in accordance with that modality which some philosophers of the mind call the *phenomenal self-model (PSM)* process of which it 'historically' becomes the actuator when "the conscious experience of being a self emerges because a large part of the PSM in your brain is transparent [...] But it can become the Ego only because you are constitutionally unable to realize that all this is just the content of a simulation in your brain" (Metzinger 2009: 7–8). From this point of view, we have "been decided" by unpredictable historical-vital movements to deal with *ourselves*, also as experienced intentional consciousnesses, by means of that causal and disordered – because it is not predetermined – evolutionary dynamic of change, so finding ourselves, quite suddenly, having re-flexive experiences with a high degree of 're-sounded' warning called *felt* and *re-felt* awareness. It is a resonance, awareness, so powerful that it can and must take on a meaning, as the 'experienced' expressive communicability 'of the surface' – language – in that it is a new living form of subjectivity even while it is pathocentric.

Here we have, therefore, the passage from a positional and static anthropology to a posthuman anthropology which implies a *"dynamic 'relational' conception of the processes of the makeup of the subject.* This subject is one which is [...] *embodied, embedded* (embedded in a living form in some environmental niche), *enacted* (involved in a performance and engaging self-representation), *extended* (ready to project itself in the performances of others), *emerging* (emerging from the whole "chaotic network of the experience), *affective* (not only cognitive) and *relational* (involved in a series of interactions with both the objects and the subjects of the world)" (Eugeni 2015: 62, 63).

Humanistic subjectivity appears to be obsolete because it emerged from an interdisciplinary approach to knowledge supported by the human body which becomes a transitive and transitory ground for relationary dialogue with the theriomorphic and technomorphic dimensions; a dialogue which is not only a constant dialogical and emotional relation but which frequently becomes an occasion for ontological hybridization. "This affirmative, unprogrammed mutation can help actualize new concepts, affects and planetary subject formations" (Braidotti 2013: 104).

On the one hand, there has been an increasing interest in corporeity which is a circular interpretation of the multiplicative expression of objectivity as a vital affective-emotive area; on the other, with the rapid and unstoppable development of biotechno-science, we must not underestimate the normalizing reductionism of performative possibilities provided by the growing area of info-quantitative computation: in the posthuman age, it is not possible to neglect traditional critical thought, which makes it necessary "to emphasize the importance of critical theory, in the sense of a mix of critique and creativity that makes it imperative for us to come to terms with the present in new, fundamental ways" (Braidotti 2013: 187).

The incessant and speedy development of technology makes us able to see the possibility of achieving the unthinkable in the posthuman age. It makes us wish for more and modifies its meaning, and favours the multiplication and acceleration of choices compared to the multiplicative investigation of possibilities which require a new affective/emotive education. The future potential that this promises is of various kinds, ranging from boundless hopes to atavistic fears, so that there is a wall between the positions of "technophobes" and "technophiles" in which a certain extreme picture of the posthuman risks resembling eugenic ideologies or science fiction (Rossi 2008). It is true that, by means of bio-technology, life is molecularised and that this has significant effects on our biological way of being and therefore on our affections: one only has to think of the possibilitities of physical and moral *Human Enhancement* through technical grafting and biochemical modification which will more and more often have a role to play in improving the character of an individual or even create physical and moral performance on demand and according to need. While the posthuman criticises modern humanistic anthropocentrism in favour of pathocentric anthropodecentrism and prefers a model of education and improvement if the affective/emotive level, enabling man to acquire more ways of expressing himself openly, creatively and interlocutively with animal and machine otherness in the construction of a *pathosophie* based on "sensitive reasoning", we are also aware that so-called other forms of posthumanism which are part of the general category, such as "hyperhumanism" and "transhumanism" (Marchesini 2002, Bostrom 2005,

Venter 2013) are forms of extreme humanistic anthropocentrism in that they wish to bring about further enhancement of human control over the world by means of forms of biotechno-political imperialism which, as well as developing a model of rational subjectivisation of the logical/arithmocrat kind, aim to become the historical and metaphysical Subject, holding absolute power over all living subjects by means of biotechnopolitical subjection with processes governed by biotechnological *Enhancement* made possible by economic and technoscientific power. Until a few decades ago, in fact, all that biomedicine could aspire to was to arrest 'abnormality', re-establish the vital 'norm' of the natural. Thanks to biotechnology, the 'normativity' and 'normativities' of the body have become open to the mutation and experiential multiplication of themselves and are in need of new biotechno-political thinking.

The old boundaries between prevention, cure, correction and 'optimization' (Balistreri 2011, Adele 2012, Tolleneer/Sterckx/Bonte 2013; Savulescu/Meulen/Kahane 2011, Buchanan 2011) need to be redrawn: think, for example, of the effects of psychiatric drugs in re-establishing "thresholds", the norms and volatility of the emotions, cognition and will (Metzinger 2009, Maturo/Barker 2012), the constant modification of female reproduction processes by multiplying forms of assisted conception, female aging modified by hormone therapy, the increasing prospect of enhanced prosthetics, the long-term prospect of 'cultivating' organs in vitro to be grafted, and the introduction of biotechnological devices by means of nanotechnology, and so on.

By means of biotechnology, in the age of the posthuman in its "hyper-humanistic" and "transhumanistic" forms, control of the living body has become essential in advanced liberal democracies and human beings have begun to interpret and experiment on themselves and their lives in terms that are fundamentally biomedical, so ending up being subjected to the assistance and judgement of biotechno-medicine. "We are increasingly coming to relate to ourselves as 'somatic' individuals, that is to say, as beings whose individuality is, in part at least, grounded within our fleshly, corporeal existence, and who experience, articulate, judge, and act upon ourselves in part in the language of biomedicine" (N. Rose 2007: 24–25). While in the nineteenth and twentieth centuries biological assumptions were already, either implicitly or explicitly, behind many ideas of what was meant by citizenship, with the inevitable threat of the spectre of racial nationalist politics, the image/idea of contemporary "biological citizenship" seems to be significantly different in the eugenic age (Esposito 2008, Agamben 1998).

The practice of genetic diagnosis, in particular in relation to the possibility of having "tailor-made" children (Agar 2006) or *saviour siblings*

(H. Rose/S. Rose 2012) invites us to significant reflection of an ethical nature, and therefore to moderate the technological optimism which are inherent in some types of the posthuman, while at the same time there is no lack of risking the development of a culture leaning towards a "genetic self-optimizing of the human species in different directions, thus jeopardizing the unity of human nature as basis, up to now, for all human beings to understand and mutually recognize one another" (Habermas 2003: 121).

Apart from the new moral responsibilities, the need for public discussion and political debate with regard to these specific questions, we should note that new languages, new aspirations and wishes and new expressions are taking shape with the posthuman "construction" of citizenship in biological and genetic terms in which biological images, explanations, values and judgements intertwine with other descriptive languages and other self-valuation criteria, significantly influenciing the perception that individuals have of themselves in terms of knowledge and practicability of their "somatic identity" (N. Rose 2007). The "biological citizen", in fact, uses biologically-enhanced languages to describe aspects of himself and his identity governed by media information which is becoming more and more invasive, and in the world of risk, of susceptibility, caution and ability to predict we see how "somatic identity" is assuming a new potential value in the construction, wholly posthuman, of "biological citizenship" both on the individual and on the collective level (Giacca/Gobbato 2010).

The "somatic individual" as such, for example, faces our decision on whether it is to be tested genetically in order to predict and programme its future, and we need to behave with caution in such circumstances in terms of procreative, employment, insurance choices, while the risk of indiscriminate use of genetic information increases (Rodotà 2004, N. Rose 2007). The collective aspect, in contrast, relates to "biosocial" groups organized around biomedical categories (Rabinow 1996). They consist of ordinary forms of activity such as public communication campaigns aimed at achieving better cures, freedom from stigma, and access to services.

"Biological citizenship", therefore, shows up in a whole series of new identities and forms of collectivization which are expressed in the demand for recognition, access to knowledge, claims to competence and the birth of "new rights" (Rodotà 2006) arising from the more general "right to health" which would be better defined as "the right of every being that is born to participate in the rich experiences of life deservingly and fully".

Since a society is organized according to ideals of health and life, in fact, biomedicine has modified what we think we have a right to hope for as well as the objectives to which we can aspire, with inevitable affective/emotive implications for the *pathei*. As a result, many "biological citizens" think they have acquired the right to treatment for their illness or disability while assuming that others – politicians, doctors and health authorities – are responsible for themselves. It is no rare matter for citizens to claim justice for their personal situation. The political authorities, on the other hand, have taken on the task and responsibility of safeguarding and strengthening the "biological capital" of the people. So large sums of money are made available for research and development, invested in healthcare by national governments and private foundations. Since the beginning of the 21st century, the overall value of biomedical biotechnology in all its derived industrial forms has become immense, and national and local politics in the world continue to promote its growth. It is patent that the reason is not simply the pursuit of health 'optimization', but also the creation of wealth.

"Bioeconomy", which is those aspects of economic activity that "have as their organizing principle the capturing of the latent value in biological processes, a value that is simultaneously that of human health and that of economic growth" (Organisation for Economic Cooperation and Development – OECD, N. Rose 2007: 32–33), is now an essential part of the global economy and has been made possible by the digitalization of biological data carried out by institutions ranging from age-old European and American scientific centres to emerging giants such as those in China, Singapore and India.

Techno-science pretends to be, and thinks that it succeeds in appearing, necessarily disinterested, a 'pure science' and democratically legitimate, but the truth is that the real driving force of scientific research is basically the profit motive, for "since the first discoveries in molecular biology that 'genetic engineering' the creation to order of genetically altered organisms, has an immense possibility for producing private profit [...] As a consequence of these possibilities, molecular biologists have become entrepreneurs. Many have founded biotechnology firms funded by venture capitalists. Some have become very rich when a successful public offering of their stock has made them suddenly the holders of a lot of valuable paper. Others find themselves with large blocks of stock in international pharmaceutical companies who have bought out the biologist's mom-and-pop enterprise and acquired their expertise in the bargain" (Lewontin 2000: 162–163). In a context in which the globalization of markets and technologies permits and, to a certain extent, imposes the circulation of all products, the production of life knowledge, which can be economically exploited, takes advantage of diverse transnational networks with the aim of mobilising and linking material artefacts, tissues, cell lines, reagents, DNA sequences, techniques, researchers, fundings, production and commercialization. But in the name of an assumed *freedom* of research, profit must not be the only motive, and it is for this reason that we have to pursue an ethical line in the posthuman age threatened by "hyperhumanist" anxiety and hallucinatory "transhumanistic" ambitions.

While it is true that "bioeconomics", an example of which is the numerous biotechnological "Human Genomics" companies, European and other, that focus on ethics and informed consent and speculate on the ethically correct treatment of human tissues and medical data, so radically changing the concept of human life and creating new value categories that penetrate market relationships, the sphere of ethics is no longer limited to the morality that governs new forms of economic exchange relating to life, but itself, by controlling this new form of economics – sales, purchase, the exploitation of tissues, cells, embryos, ovums, sperm, body parts – becomes in its turn a legitimized "saleable resource" (N. Rose 2007, H. Rose/S. Rose 2012).

With advances in technoscientific developments, those aspects of life which were once thought to be in the hands of "fate" have become the object of decision and deliberation, so constituting a new *"bioanthropotechincal* ethics" (Masullo 2011: 87), or ethics of the posthuman, in the transitional stage towards a new image of man biologically and technologically conceived, an image which is threatened by "hyperhumanistic" and "transhumanistic" models.

Man himself, repositioning himself in the natural world, has an opportunity, perhaps for the first time in the story of life, to be at least partly *determined* and "oriented" by himself and not only as the *Bios* but also as the *Zoe*. Man becomes a conscious transformative process: for the first time as an abstract subject, in one way rooted *in* a nature which has moulded *him*, in another way separated from it and therefore from his *dominus* which has "forced" him to construct the reassuring but illusory defence of "second nature", in which he has placed his *logos* and his Ego as "Absolute Lords" on the model of humanistic anthropocentrism, now, having really become *homo creator* (Scheler 1915) and for this reason too postuma, he has an opportunity, in spite of the risks involved, to influence the process of mutation of the self to his originary constitution (form). In this possibility of *decision* and the condition of being himself the only agent of change, being natural and at the same time "super-natural" (that is, the continuer of nature *beyond* – also *within* – nature itself, lies the new ethicals condition we have named *bioanthropotechnical*.

In this new prospect of the posthuman scenario, then, there is no lack of posthuman *bioanthropotechical* ethical considerations which might now actively contribute to *making the human posthuman*, given the life and the potential it has. It is therefore possible to claim that "to the biological citizen, as a new form of the species, is given the task of inter-pretor of the 'necessity' of mutation of the form of man" and the human capacity to "overcome the old limitations, which have now become *performative* 'thresholds' by means of technological integration." (Masullo 2011: 88).

In the age of the molecular biopolitics of life, the "biological citizen" is required to evaluate, judge and ethically justify decisions regarding human life and not only, in a context of somatic "reconfiguration" and "reprogramming" which makes us inquire "about the future not so much of our being as much as our becoming: a 'new becoming' of men, the living, the world." (Masullo 2008: 6).

If biotechnological mutation proves able to keep to the anthropocen-trative and patho-centric model of the posthuman and does not take on forms of further hyperhumanistic anthropocentrism or, worse, of "a-pathic" transhumanist technocentrism, it will probably be gradual rather than revolutionary, continuative rather than epoch-making, and most of the changes that take place in clinical and therapeutic procedures will soon become an integral part of our way of life, of thinking and behaving.

Therefore, by avoiding the disquieting apocalypticism of the "techno-phobes" and the illusory dreamlike predictions of the "technophylics" the posthuman "biological citizen" should be looked at not accompanied by the question "What is the human being?" but thinking about what kind of image we wish to keep of the human being, given that it has become possible to "improve" it; and thinking of what aspects we wish to *take care of* in order to avoid the risk of *losing the world* and to ensure both for ourselves and future generations a "satisfying life", "a life worth of living" (Pulcini 2004: 34; Jonas 1994; Anders 2002a, 2002b).

The posthuman condition as an emerging 'fact' of the intrusion of "bio-techno-computer" procedures opens up political reflections on the tightrope of whether it should be regarded as the politics *about* or poli-tics *of* life (Esposito 2008), with its constant wavering between the promotion of life and of health and its negation, between *biotechnology* as an organised system of instrumental support at the service of life and health and reduction to a *techne* of the *bios* as "technocracy", as an a-pathic "technical system" (see Ellul 2004) which, in a "technophilic" prospective entrusts to technology "the destiny of man to be enslaved" (Masullo 2011: 84) in a time of development of the overwhelming ideological violence of technology *over* the living. The anthropology of the posthuman, then, should be conceived of in the perspective of a *bio-anthropo-technology* which, by being based on the hybridative processes of both *bios* and *techne*, seems to be a possible and reasonable form of 'development' of the living-man which promotes the *techne* without neglecting the *bios*, offering possibilities of a more open etheroriperal experiential interlocution between discrete states of multiple and practicable individual patho-centric subjectivities.

With the emergence of the posthuman condition, therefore, "it is not only man's *ownership* of his animality that is at stake, but also his increasing tendency to *take responsibility for it* through the use of technology." (Fimiani 2005: 119).

While, on the one hand, the posthuman condition is taking us in great strides towards the age of the "biological citizen" and even more so towards that of the "bio-technological citizen", which includes not only the social and political dimension of the structuring of "new forms of existence" but also the emergence of opportunities for new forms of affective experience of life, on the other our additional interface with machines is developing "other" affective sensibilities and perspectives which intersect and modify modes of feeling and behaving which require vigilant awareness.

The revolution brought about by the birth of biology and the increasingly powerful human ability to understand and control it, to the extent of 'reinventing' it, above all by means of the recent development of biotechnologies, means that posthuman anthropology has to ask new questions not about the essence of man, but about his becoming and his ability to "make himself become" by designing himself, definitely not "creating himself", on the basis of an asset which, now emptied of its essence, is obscure, just as his own possible destiny is obscure, even threatened, by his own doing, with being removed from being a significant patho-centric experience of present-day history and "added" to those many senseless events that have marked and are marking the story of life as an integral opportunity, within the cosmic silence, of "affective necessity".

Note

1   The term *Pathosophie* was used as the title of one of the main works of the German neurophysiologist and philosopher Viktor von Weizsäcker (1886–1957), *Pathosophie* (1955) (Weizsäcker 2005). More in general, from 1930 von Weizsäcker introduced the term *pathisch* to describe the antilogical (*antilogik*) character of life *tout court*, and of the human being in particular, with the object of addressing the "bottomless bottom" of life in its general

relationship with emotional life, described as the "basic relationship" (*Grund-Verhältnis*) which is obscure and unobjectifiable.

Seen from this point of view, action and knowledge, animal and human, are primarily dependent on the affections. Starting from this assumption, the cited work by von Weizsäcker develops a "theory of the affections" in an attempt to understand human nature and behavior, based on our mutual natural identity with the *animal* and the specific degree of our condition as a living *patiens* being.

The basic aim of Weizsäcker's theory of the affections is the recognition and classification of the range of our basic emotions as they are found in the meanings of the five German auxiliary modal verbs: *Können* (be able to), *Wollen* (will), *Müssen* (must), *Dürfen* (be allowed to), and *Sollen* (have to). Here, the specific human element compared to other living beings with whom the human being shares the first four *pathe* – though with a very different import and intensity – is the fifth modal verb, *Sollen* (moral obligation). Weizsäcker named these five modal verbs, as applied to the affective basis of man's life, *pathisches Pentagramm*.

Bibliography

Adele, C. 2012: *A Guide to Human Enhancement Including its Purpose, Existing technologies, Emerging Technologies, Speculative Technologies and More*. Kansas: Webster's Digital Services.

Agamben, G. 1998: *Homo sacer. Sovereign Power and Bare Life*, trans. D. Heller-Roazen. Stanford: Stanford University Press.

Agar, N. 2006: Designer Babies: Ethical Considerations. *ActionBioscience*, April 2006.

Anders, G. [1956] 2002a: *Die Antiquiertheit des Menschen 1. Über die Seele im Zeitalter der zweiten industriellen Revolution*. München: Beck.

Anders, G. [1980] 2002b: *Die Antiquiertheit des Menschen 2. Über die Zerstörung des Lebens im Zeitalter der dritten industriellen Revolution*. München: Beck.

Balistreri, M. 2011: *Superumani. Etica ed enhancement*. Torino: Espress Edizioni.

Bodei, R. 2004: *Destini personali. L'età della colonizzazione delle coscienze*. Milano: Feltrinelli.

Borgogna, P. 2005: *Sociologia del corpo*. Roma-Bari Laterza.

Bostrom, N. 2005: A History of Transhumanist Thought, *Journal of Evolution and Technology* XIV (1), 1–25.

Braidotti, R. 1994: *Nomadic Subjects. Embodiment and Sexual Difference in Contemporary Feminist Theory*. New York: Columbia University Press.

Braidotti, R. 2013: *The Posthuman*. Cambridge: Polity Press.

Brockman, J. 2003: *The New Humanists. Science at the Edge*. New York: Barnes & Noble.

Buchanan, A. 2011: *Better than Human: The Promise and Perils of Enhancing Ourselves*. Oxford: Oxford University Press.

Deleuze, G., Guattari, F. [1972] 2000: *Anti-Oedipus. Capitalism and Schizophrenia*, trans. R. Hurley *et al*. Minneapolis: University of Minnesota Press.

Deleuze, G. / Guattari, F. [1980] 2005: *A Thousand Plateaus. Capitalism and Schizophrenia*, trans. B. Massumi. Minneapolis/London: University of Minnesota Press.

Denton, D. 2005: *Les émotions primordiales et l'éveil de la conscience*. Paris: Flammarion.

Esposito, R. 2008: *Bíos. Biopolitics and Philosophy*, trans. Th. Campbell. Minneapolis/London: University of Minnesota Press.

Ellul, J. 1980: *The Technological System*, trans. J. Neugroschel. New York: Continuum.

Eugeni, R. 2015: *La condizione postmediale. Media, linguaggi e narrazioni*. Brescia: La Scuola.

Fimiani, M. 2005: *Antropologia filosofica*. Roma: Editori Riuniti.

Gehlen A. [1940] 1988: *Man. His Nature and Place in the World*, trans. C. McMillan and K. Pillemer. New York: Columbia University Press.

Giacca, M., Gobbato, C. A. (eds) 2010: *Salute e Società* IX (3) (*Polis genetica e società del futuro*).

Guzzardi, L. (ed.) 2015: *Il pensiero acentrico. L'irruzione del caos nell'impresa conoscitiva*. Milano: elèuthera.

Habermas, J. 2003: *The Future of Human Nature*, trans. M. Pensky *et al.*, Cambridge: Polity.

Haraway, D. 2008: *When Species Meet*. Minneapolis: University of Minnesota Press. Herbrechter, S. 2009: *Postumanismus*. Frankfurt am Main: Surkamp.

Jonas, H. 1984: *The Imperative of Responsibility: In Search of Ethics for the Technological Age*, trans. H. Jonas and D. Herr. Chicago/London: University of Chicago Press.

Kurzweil, R. 2005: *Singularity is Near*. New York: Viking Press.

Lanza, R., Berman, B. 2009: *Biocentrism*. Dallas: BenBella Books.

Lewontin, R. 2001: *It Ain't Necessarily So: The Dream of the Human Genome and Other Illusions*. New York: New York Review of Books.

Marchesini, R. 2002: *Post-human. Verso nuovi modelli di esistenza*. Torino: Bollati Boringhieri.

Marchesini, R. 2014: Alla fonte di Epimeteo. *aut aut* 361 (*La condizione postumana*), 34–51.

Masullo, P. A. 2008: *L'umano in transito. Saggio di antropologia filosofica*. Bari: Edizioni di Pagina.

Masullo, P. A. 2011: *Critica della salute bioantropotecnica*. "Teoria" XXXI (1), 81–92.

Masullo, P. A. 2014: *Il patico come modo essenziale della "forma-vita"*. "Thaumazein" 2 (*Critica della ragione medica*), 433–454.

Maturo, A., Barker, K. K. (eds) 2012: *La medicina delle emozioni e delle cognizioni*. "Salute e Società" XI (2).

Mayr, E. 1982: *The Growth of Biological Thought. Diversity, Evolution and Inheritance*. Cambridge (MA)/London: Belknap Press.

Mayr, E. 2004: *What Makes Biology Unique? Considerations on the Autonomy of a Scientific Discipline*. Cambridge: Cambridge University Press.

Metzinger, T. 2009: *The Ego Tunnel. The Science of the Mind and the Myth of the Self*. New York: Basic Books.

Nietzsche, F. 1873: On Truth and Lying in a Non-Moral Sense. In *The Birth of Tragedy and Other Writings,* trans. R. Guess and R. Speirs. Cambridge: Cambridge University Press 2007, 139–153.

Nietzsche, F. 2006: *Writings from the Late Notebooks,* trans. R. Bittner. Cambridge: Cambridge University Press.

Pfänder, A. 1911: *Motive und Motivation.* In A. Pfänder (ed.), *Münchener Philosophische Abhandlungen. Festschrift für Theodor Lipps.* Leipzig: Barth, 163–195.

Plessner, H. 1981: Die Stufen des Organischen und der Mensch. Einleitung in die philosophische Anthropologie. In *Gesammelte Schriften IV,* hrsg. von G. Dux *et al.* Frankfurt am Main: Suhrkamp 1981.

Pulcini, E. 2004: L'«homo creator» e la perdita del mondo. In E. Pulcini, M. Fimiani, V. G. Kurotschka (eds), *Umano Post-Umano. Potere, sapere, etica nell'età globale.* Roma: Editori Riuniti, 11–41.

Rabinow, P. 1996: Artificiality and Enlightenment: From Sociobiology to Biosociality. In *Essays on the Anthropology of Reason.* Princeton: Princeton University Press, 234–252.

Roden, D. 2014: *Posthuman Life: Philosophy at the Edge of the Human.* London/New York: Routledge.

Rodotà, S. 2004: *Tecnopolitica. La democrazia e le nuove tecnologie della comunicazione* (nuova edizione accresciuta). Roma-Bari: Laterza.

Rodotà, S. 2006: *La vita e le regole. Tra diritto e non diritto.* Milano: Feltrinelli.

Rose, H., Rose, S. 2012: *Genes, Cells and Brains. The Promethean Promises of New Biology.* London /New York: Verso.

Rose, N. 2007: *The Politics of Life Itself. Biomedicine, Power and Subjectivity in the Twenty-First Century.* Princeton: Princeton University Press.

Rossi, P. 2008: *Speranze.* Bologna: il Mulino.

Savulescu, J., Meulen, R., Kahane, G. (eds) 2011: *Enhancing Human Capacities.* Oxford: Oxford University Press.

Scheler, M. [1928] 2009: *The Human Place in the Cosmos,* trans. M. Frings. Evanston (Illinois): Northwestern University Press.

Scheler, M. 1915: On the Idea of Man. *Journal of the British Society for Phenomenology* IX (3) 1978, 184–198.

Schiavone, A. 2007: *Storia e destino.* Torino: Einaudi.

Simondon, G. 2005: *L'individuation à la lumière des notions de forme et d'information.* Grenoble: Millon.

Spinoza, B. [1677] 2002: *Ethics.* In *Complete Works,* edited by M. L. Morgan. Indianapolis/Cambridge: Hackett, 213–382.

Tolleneer, J., Sterckx, S., Bonte, P. (eds) 2013: *Athletic Enhancement, Human Nature and Ethics.* Dordrecht: Kluwer.

Venter, C. J. 2013: *Life at the Speed of Light. From the Double Helix to the Dawn of Digital Life.* New York: Viking.

Weizsäscker, V. von 2005: *Gesammelte Schriften Band 10. Pathosophie,* hrsg. von W. Schindler u.a. Frankfurt am Main: Surkamp.

Wolfe, C. 2010: *What is Post_Humanism?* Minneapolis: University of Minnesota Press.

CHAPTER

9

The Stratification of Empathic Experience

ANNA DONISE

Studies of decisional processes have been considerably carried forward by experimental research over the past fifty years. While, for a long time, analyses of decision and, in particular, its moral evaluation have focused on the role of rationality and demonstrated its significance (see, for example, Kohlberg/Turiel 1971), since the eighties increasingly more attention has been paid to the role of the emotional sphere. Numerous studies have investigated the role of the emotions in decision making traditionally thought of as being 'rational' (Damasio 1995) or the way in which our moral judgments vary according to whether situations are personal or impersonal (see on this subject: Greene 2001, 2004 and 2009). In Greene's version of the "Duel-process theory", it is hypothesized that both superior cognitive processes and immediate emotive processes are involved, and that the different responses to these apparently similar questions depend on the way in which one process prevails over the other. Greene and his team have used functional magnetic resonance (fMRI) to monitor which cerebral areas are involved in reasoning which lead to decisions, so demonstrating that different areas are activated in different situations. In particular, the resumed use of so-called "trolley problems" (Foot 1967, Thompson 1976) has produced what is now called "trolleyology" (see Edmonds 2013). In the simplest version of the predicament, we have two similar questions posed in relation to an initial situation: a trolley is about to run into and kill five people working on the rails. In one case, thanks to a lever, the trolley's path can be deviated onto a rail where there is only one worker; in the other, however, one has to decide whether to throw onto the rails a fat man whose body would divert the trolley and save the five workers. From the point of view of costs/benefits the alternatives are equal: one man dies in order to save five. But our personal involvement is very different and consequently the responses given by the subjects involved in the experiments to the two alternatives are different. Analyses carried out thanks to a neuroimaging system shows that, in the case if the reasoning that calls for our personal and physical involvement (physically throw the fat man from the bridge and kill him) are activated by those areas of the brain that are involved in the interpretation of the thoughts and feelings of *others*. When our reasoning brings others close to ourselves, the type of response and decision varies greatly. Our capacity to feel what others feel or to "put ourselves in their shoes" determines a completely different attitude in the subject who is judging or choosing: almost nobody says he is prepared to kill the fat man.

This capacity – called "empathy" only since 1909 by Titchener, who uses a neologism (from the Greek *empatheia*) to express in English the German "*Einfühlung*" (see Titchener 1909) – is an interesting way of beginning an investigation of the emotive sphere and, more generally, of the human; especially if one bears in mind that it is experimental study of the neurobiological basis of empathy that enables us the rethink the human and his ethical dimension, not according to the traditional dichotomy of reason versus emotion, but rather in relation to an intertwining of the body–mental dimension, seen as systems which are biologically, psychologically and phenomenologically integrated (Boella 2011: 104). Research into empathy is not limited, therefore, to describing our way of relating to others, but also tells us much about what makes us tick, so contributing to a definition of those characteristics that are more properly ours.

As I intend to show in the pages which follow, our capacity to enter into relation with the experience of others, that is to be empathic subjects, is not simply an emotion; it can be associated neither with primary emotions such as joy, fear or disgust, nor with secondary ones (or moral emotions, see Haidt 2003) such as shame, pride or gratitude. That is, empathy cannot be confused with "sympathy" because empathy is a way of being in the world of man – it involves every shade of emotion, from compassion to cruelty – and has its roots in our prereflexive and original makeup. Research into empathy enables us to understand, as if from some kind of privileged observatory, the structural weaving of the emotive and cognitive dimension, clearly showing the impossibility of separating the two unless for purposes of methodological abstraction. Long before we are capable of reflecting and theorizing the experience of others, in an innate way we map the movements of others through our own kinesthetic sensations (Gopnik/Meltzoff 1997). By the end of the first years of life, babies show understanding of the intentions and attitudes of others towards themselves; this does not involve mentalization and may be defined "primary intersubjectivity" (Gallagher/Zahavi 2008: 187–189). It is clear, however, that secondary intersubjectivity, which implies consciousness of the fact that the other individual, with his own aims, desires and point of view about things (therefore the acquisition of a "theory of mind", see Baron-Cohen/ Leslie/Frith 1985) cannot be reached with the immediate instinctive stage connected to the bodily dimension.

This subject was researched in the early twentieth century in the tradition straddling psychology and philosophy (see Lipps 1906, Stern 1897, Geiger 1911), but it was the phenomenological tradition which dedicated a wide range of studies to empathy (Husserl 1989, Stein 1964); in particular, Max Scheler underlines the importance of the characteristic stratification of empathic experience. And I feel it is useful to refer to Scheler in our wish to highlight some central points in reflecting on the role of empathy in ethics. His anthropological analysis gives us useful theoretical tools, in particular:

1. to identify the different levels of empathic relation: from the fusional and instinctive to those which admit of separation between each other, to the more cognitive levels which imply "putting ourselves in the other's shoes".
2. to recognise that admitting the role of emotions in judgement and in particular in ethical judgement does not mean maintaining that the emotive or empathic dimension mechanically determine our behaviour, or that they are sufficient for the definition of correct behaviour.

1. The Body as an Expressive Field

The first problem that one encounters in investigating empathy is its definition. "Empathy" is first and foremost the capacity to feel the experience of another. However, I can see his body but I do not have direct access to what his consciousness experiences. The only experience I have direct access to is my own. Much of modern thought has looked at the intersubjective relation on the basis of the assumption that my experience, insofar as it is mine, can be acknowledged because of its immediate presence. As for the external world, the subject might be mistaken, and his own experience is the only thing he can be sure of. Max Scheler urges us not to accept unquestioningly that "inner perception, as opposed to the external perception of nature, can never deceive"

(Scheler 1973: 3). If it is true, in fact, that our perception of the external world can be the cause of illusions and erroneous judgment, an appropriate investigation will tell us that also our relation to the experiences of our consciousness might deceive us. A stick immersed in water appears to be broken, but looking at our authentic intentions might also be difficult; often, in fact, we deceive ourselves by removing or masking the real motive for an action.[1] Our psychic life is much less transparent than we think.

Our point of view is, shall we say, turned upside-down: in contesting the supremacy of the pure interiority of consciousness, we rehabilitate the cognitive value of action towards the external world. An important part of this rehabilitation is linked to the emotive sphere, which tells us a great deal about the world in which we find ourselves. When meeting another person, I am aware of his expressions, his way of talking, walking and blushing: basically, I am aware of his living body as an expressive field of his experiences. In line with Husserl's idea, Scheler gives great significance to this concept of the *living body*, contesting the idea that "after all, we are given only the body". The body of the other is never perceptibly "a dead organic body" or a *Körper* to which something like a psychic experience is added; on the contrary, we are primarily aware of the expressions of the living body or *Leib* (see Husserl 1989, 1977). This immediacy does not imply that we might not be mistaken about the other's experience, but error is a possibility not to be excluded even for my own interior experience. In its expression, which becomes the keystone for reflection on intersubjectivity (Boella 2010), I encounter the experience of the other but it is given to me immediately and clearly: in his blushing I see embarrassment, in a gesture, anger. I am not aware of the body or of the psyche, but of "integral wholes" (Scheler 2008: 257; see Masullo 2013). This is a constitutive level preceding the reflexive dimension: so it is not necessary – and here we distance ourselves from Husserl – to hypothesize a similarity between me and the other that enables us, on the basis of our own experience, to see the other, by analogy, as *alter ego*. On the contrary, the centrality attributed to the body, which becomes a constitutive principle of experience, must be recognized by both sides of the relation: knowledge of ourselves is not a purely mental process, nor does it exist in a condition of isolation from others. The relation of my body to the environment establishes a world of possibility or *affordances* (see Gibson 1986) which, together with what my body forbids or restricts, defines the possible or the impossible (Husserl 1989: 269–288); a surrounding world which in relation to my corporeity becomes a set of "situations of meaning and circumstances for action" (Gallagher/Zahavi 2008: 138).

On the other hand, also in our relations with others we should not think – at least at the original pre-reflexive level – of an inferential nature relation. In seeing the body of another, I do not see it without its expression: "I can tell from the expressive 'look' of a person whether he is well or ill disposed towards me, long before I can tell what colour or size his eyes may be" (Scheler 2008: 240).

In Scheler's view, the assumption of the superiority of perception of internal experience is the origin of many errors in describing the inter-subjective relation. From a sufficient analysis of the human it would emerge that in the constitutive and original phase of the human being "What occurs, rather, is an immediate flow of experiences, *indifferenti-ated as between mine and thine,* which actually contains not our own and others' experiences intermingled and without distinction from one another" (Scheler 2008: 242).

2. Unipathy

This unique and undifferentiated flow of experiences cannot be considered as any real relation to the other because it occurs at moments in which there is no longer or there is not yet any individualization and separation between I and you. The clearest unipathic moments are those which connect to the origin of our history from a point of view which is both phylogenetic and ontogenetic. The "primitive psychic life of peoples", like "the facts of psychic life in infancy", show that the single individual with his feelings, his ideas and his thoughts, emerges only at a certain point of development (on this subject see Jaynes 2000). But the fusional and unipathic dimension is not abandoned once infancy is over because it is rooted, according to Scheler, in our "vital consciousness", a psychic, impulsive and instinctive dimension that must be distinguished both from the personal spirit and from the bodily dimension. Unipathic experiences exist, that is, halfway between spirit and nature (Volkelt 1876, see Wagner 2014), they are constitutive of the human being and have to do with the vital dimension. The vital element is felt and recognized in every organic movement, different from the inorganic. In fact, progressive acquisition in development does not involve psychic or vital components in a body which was earlier recognized as being inanimate; on the contrary, the movement is inverse: "Learning, in this sense, is not animation, but continual *'deanimation'*" (Scheler 2008: 235). It is only from the unipathic dimension, which is the vital, instinctive, unconscious and impulsive foundation, that spiritual life can emerge. The unipathic flow is a kind of primitive basis for the development of more, it is a unique feeling which precedes the distinction between I and you (see Cusinato 2012).

Unipathy, as a vital and primordial element, does not belong only to man, but can be seen also in much of animal behaviour. We can speak of unipathy, for example, in relation to the ability of the wasp to immobilize spiders, beetles and caterpillars with a sting that does not kill. Wasps paralyze caterpillars with great precision, and this leads us to hypothesize a kind of identification of the vital flow of the wasp with the vital process and organism of the caterpillar (Scheler 2008: 24–25, Bergson 1944: 168). The sure instinct which guides the wasp can be interpreted as "an abnormal increase" of the genuine unipathy which characterizes certain human relations. After all, it is because of this animal, instinctive and unipathic dimension that man develops in the progressive emergence of self-consciousness and individuality. In this sense "gregariousness in animals represents an advance toward the human level_whereas man becomes more of an animal by associating himself with the crowd, and more of a man by cultivating his spiritual independence" (Scheler 2008: 35; here the basic reference is to Nietzsche 2008).

In attempting to construct a true phenomenology of unipathic fusion, we can isolate three forms which are greatly different from each other:

1. *Phylogentic unipathy*. We can speak of this kind of fusion when the way of feeling relates to the origins of man's history; certain religious cults of primitive peoples seem to assume an identification of man with the totemic animal, or even with the animated totemic object (Lévy-Bruhl 1921). Also the identification of the individual with an ancestor, a real identification by which he, in being alive here and now *is* at the same time one of his ancestors ("he is not merely like his ancestor, or guided and ruled by him, but actually *is*, in his present life, at the same time one of his ancestors", Scheler 2008: 15), is a unipathic relation which from an historical point of view is that which is defined the "ancestor cult". This cult, in fact, represents a form of ritualization and therefore a liberation and overcoming of the effective unipathic relation: necessarily present in ritualization is the consciousness of diversity between man and his ancestors (see Frobenius 1921).

2. *Ontogenetic unipathy*. A clear case of unipathy which we all, or almost all, experience is the relation between mother and child. This bond is often interpreted as a radical form of love, so that it becomes a kind of test of theories which define love as the capacity to accept the other as part of the self (Hartmann 1869). Scheler upturns this idea and maintains, on the contrary, that in the unipathy between mother and child there exists, in its attitude of dedication, a kind of identification of the mother with the ego of the child. The maternal instinct is a form of unipathy because it allows the mother to deeply feel – in a fusional way, indeed – the needs of the newborn baby; "The rhythm of lactation and milk-tension in the ring hunger, which likewise holds between the satisfaction afforded to the mother by suckling and to the child by taking the breast [...] The intuitive *psycho-somatic-unity* of mother and child is not so entirely severed by their physical separation" (Scheler 2008: 23). When the baby is very young, the unipathic instinct allows for constant care and harmonic development.

However, it is in maintaining the organic development of the baby, with care and attention, that the maternal instinct might block and even prevent psychic and spiritual development; the mother holds the baby close to her, almost as if wanting "to draw the child back" (Scheler 2008: 23). So there is no real continuity between unipathic instinct and maternal love; quite the opposite, instinct and love are often in conflict with each other: love, even real maternal love, can come into being only if the unipathic and fusional tendency is overcome so that the baby is allowed the formation of progressively autonomous individuality; we can, in fact, talk of 'love' only when two different egos are involved in the relation.[2] Because the baby is concerned with his own progressive becoming an autonomous individual, it experiences fusional and unipathic relations more easily. In role-play, the game of 'as if', the role taken on can become, at certain moments for the baby, a reality or a quasi-reality (on this subject, see the opposing views of Bettelheim 1989 and Harris 2000). The baby girl, for example, identifies with her mother when she plays at being mother with her doll, but – but the dynamic is the same – she might react quite differently from an adult when watching a play or when listening to a fairy story.

3. *Unipathic phenomena in everyday life*. Lastly, it is important to recognise that unipathy is not linked exclusively to the origin dimension. On the contrary, unipathic fusion, naturally and with various gradation, is it manifested in many moments of the psychic life of the adult. Scheler is interested in studies – which were numerous in his time – of hypnosis (Schilder 1922). In the hypnotic relation, the characteristics of the primitive ego and of the child's ego are artificially reproduced in the person hypnotized. In authentic primitive unipathy there was, in any case, a genuine identification of existence between two egos, while in the hypnotic relation it is the spiritual centre of noetic events that is disactivated in the hypnotized patient, while the vital-automatic system is increased. "The judgment, will and choice of the subject, his love and his hate, are then no longer his own but those of the hypnotist, whose intellect is mounted, so to speak, on the back of the subject's reflex-system" (Scheler 2008: 17). The unipathic dynamic that we find in hypnosis, therefore, has to do with a kind of spiritual control which can be found also in psychic modalities of very common relation: passive obedience and masochism are examples. The submissive, servile subject is identified as the strong because he has pleasure in being so; this identification has the unconscious aim of coming into possession of a part of his overall strength. A similar mechanism is that which occurs in sado-masochist polarity: "Even for the masochist, the object of enjoyment is not pure passivity as such, but his self identifying participation in the dominance of the partner, i.e. a *sympathetic attainment of power*" (Scheler 2008: 18).

Unipathy manifests itself clearly also in certain forms of psychic pathology, from the hysteria analyzed by Freud (1990), which seems more like emotional contagion, to some forms of schizophrenia, in which the patient is able to identify with the personality of another, whether historical or not (see Österreich 1910).

In the analysis of present unipathic experiences, we find some forms of unipathy which might be defined forms of "reciprocal fusion" in which one ego does not prevail over the other. This is the "sexual act carried out for love" in which both parties are in a unique vital flow which contains nothing of the individual egos involved, without this entailing consciousness of "us" as a sum of the two identities. Scheler gives great importance to the sexual act and to eroticism. "The loving sexual act discloses, not knowledge indeed, but a source of possible knowledge, and metaphysical knowledge at that, which he can otherwise obtain only very imperfectly [...] or not at all." (Scheler 2008: 105). Fusional empathy, however, is not limited to the erotic sphere, but is found also in the psychic life of the masses. Non-organized masses find themselves in a state of reciprocal fusion of its members, "into a *single* stream of instinct and feeling, whose pulse thereafter governs the behaviour of all its members" (Scheler 2008: 21). Living a unipathic experience, for example the experience of being part of the crowd, takes man back into a "primordial" dimension which allows him to overcome his individual corporeity and at the same time to be "deposing and disabling" from that spiritual and intellectual individuality which makes him a subject in the full sense of the term. The example given by Scheler to clarify this point is extremely interesting, especially if one thinks that his description of it was written in 1922: "If there is any one thing within recent experience which serves to confirm these observations, it is the experience of the (First) World War. However it comes about, and whoever is to blame for it. A war-situation transforms all 'organic communities', i.e. groups and individuals having a sense of unity in their collective mode of life, into real entities of unitary and powerful kind" (Scheler 2008: 31–32). This process has effects of great significance: on the one hand, in fact, it makes the individual a hero who has raised himself above his bodily dimension so that he is less fearful for his physical safety; on the other, it "disables" his personal spirituality by reducing his level of individual awareness and responsibility. The crows is transformed into a single collective action in which both the corporal and the spiritual ego are lost.

So unipathic fusion has very precise characteristics which make it different from the empathic or sympathetic relation to another subject. Genuine unipathy, as we have seen, is automatic and is never a voluntary act, it is not chosen; even if we can identify laws or causal connections which trigger it, it is always a question of connections which have to do with "the causality of the vital" and not with motivational laws which allow us to understand connections between noetic or spiritual acts. Furthermore, it is a causality which cannot even be compared with the kind of mechanical causality which repeats itself uniformly and constantly. It is rather a causality characterised not only by a form of automatism, but also by a "tendency toward the goal" which is not to be confused with an activity which is consciously directed. A causality in which the whole of the past, and not only the immediately previous causes, is concretely in act. These characteristics of "vital causality", however, are present only if for some reason, they are deprived, at least momentarily, of certain immediately essential items of subjectivity: the sphere of personal noetic events on the one hand (that is, the spiritual dimension) and the bodily sphere of feeling and sensation on the other (the immediately body dimension with its immediate needs). Only if these two sphere are suspended can man live unipathic moments; "he must abandon his spiritual dignity and allow his instinctive life to look after itself" (Scheler 2008: 31).

3. Inhabited by Others

In our study of the masses, we shall not only experiment unipathy, but also relations which are less fusional and radical, such as emotional infection. To clarify what emotional infection involves, it is enough to think, for example, of when we go to a party simply to get over a bad mood; or when we feel great sadness, we realise "only by inference and reasoning" that our sadness was a mood of only by inference from causal considerations does it become clear where it came from. "Thus one may only notice afterwards that a mournful feeling, encountered in oneself,

is traceable to infection from group one has visited some hours before."
(Scheler 2008: 11). In general, we speak of infection when, even if there
is no intention to participate in the mood of others, and without having
any interest at all in their joy, sadness or anger, we too happen to feel
happy, sad or angry.

The unipathic dimension and that of emotional infection are similar
in that they are fusional experiences in which it is difficult or even
impossible to distinguish the experiences belonging to one's ego. Our
feelings are not always our own, in fact; many of the ideas we express,
the plans we make and judgments and opinions that we have, belong
to others, but we are inhabited by them. We grow up with others and
live in an environment that we have become a part of: we live 'first and
foremost' in the modes of feeling typical of our environment, our parents, family, and teachers (Scheler 1912: 65). Before feeling our real
sentiments, before having independent feelings of our own, we live in
a feeling "which corresponds to the direction of feeling typical of our
narrower or wider society and its tradition" (*ibid.*). Many of my feelings, by tastes and attitudes are not mine, therefore, but first and
foremost belong to the community of which I am a part. And when I
convince myself that my feelings are my own, that it is I myself who
wants certain things, to behave and judge in a particular way, I am living an illusion. "The natural direction of illusion is not that of taking
one's own for the other's or of 'emotional projecting' oneself into other
person, but the opposite, namely, *taking the other's for one's own*"
(*ibid.*). This is a tendency which is particularly characteristic of modern
consciousness, but which expresses itself only at a certain point of our
development. We can and must escape from this illusion, even if "a
long and critical confrontation is always necessary before we can make
our *own* feelings clear behind these feelings we vicariously reproduce"
(*ibid.*). In the evolutionary process, however, which coincides with progressive identification, man conquers and develops a series of rational
abilities which characterize him as an individual and as a spiritual person. At the same time, however, he loses some of his emotional and
fusional capacity until he risks what Scheler calls "hypertrophy of his
'intellect'" (Scheler 2008: 27), which is typical of modernity and in
particular of western man. The character of individual identity implies
separation, the loss of the instinctive capacity to feel in a fusional way.
This loss should not, however, be thought of as being absolute and
even civilized man must acquire awareness of always being inhabited
by the other. The human being must not be considered an individuality
locked up in itself.

4. Separating I from You

In the stratification of emotional life, it is unipathy that is the foundation which acts as the basis for a new kind of relation, that of "reproduced, vicarious feeling" (*nach-fühlen*). While unipathy is unconscious, automatic and linked to vital consciousness, the next level is born with the establishment of awareness of separation of the self from others. "We can begin to raise our own spiritual head [...] out of the stream of the emotional tradition of society" (Scheler 1973: 65) and acquire the ability to recognize certain experiences which inhabit it as belonging to another and to the context in which it exists. This second level of intersubjective relation can be conceived of by using the term "empathy": by "reliving" we mean the ability to feel the experience of others after it has been experienced by himself. This feeling is dependent on the feeling that precedes it, that of the other, and is accompanied by awareness of a separation. Feeling the suffering of others or knowing that the anger we feel belongs to the other is a basic capacity for establishing relations. The relevance of this emerges clearly when we examine pathological forms which invalidate this capacity. We can, in fact, be "deaf" to the experiences of others, as happens with depressed subjects, who concentrate on their own experience and are unreceptive to that of others; or, as recent studies show, certain forms of autism might be connected to an inability to relive the experiences of others that is, inadequate functioning of mirror neurons (see Gallese 2006); for example, those who are affected with Asperger syndrome have scarce activation of cerebral circuits controlling empathic relation (Baron-Cohen 2011).

It is very important, however, not to confuse this ability to feel the other with a real feeling together with another (*mit-fühlen*), which can be compared with "sympathy". Being able to feel the experience of others does not mean in fact, necessarily sympathizing with such experience. We might be able to feel what others feel without, however, being willing to show interest in their experiences. This has nothing to do with any pathological form, nor any kind of disability which makes it impossible to feel for the other; on the contrary, we might have a strong empathic capacity without having any sympathetic capacity. The suffering of others might leave us indifferent or it might be so big a responsibility that it makes us refuse and turn out back on it. Without considering that in the case of separation between our own experience and that of the other might not be clear, we might feel literally invaded, for example, by the suffering of the other. Finally, it might happen that those in possession of excellent empathetic capacity might feel the pain and suffering of others perfectly, in particular those that he himself has caused. This is so with he who feel joy in "tormenting" and the agony of his victim. "As he feels, vicariously, the increasing pain or suffering of his victim, so his own primary pleasure and enjoyment at the other's pain also increases" (Scheler 2008: 10). This subject is what we call the "sadist", the person who finds pleasure in making others suffer and thanks to his capacity to feel the experience of others is particularly skilful at tormenting: he knows full well where and how to inflict suffering.

Obviously such behaviour is not the exclusive prerogative of the subject affected by a psychic pathology or in the unlikely event of cruelty. Each of us is indifferent and sadistic, brutal and empathetic, cruel and sympathetic at the same time and knowing what others feel can sometimes be a valuable instrument to inflict the worst kinds of suffering: we have all used, and use every day, our capacity for empathy to welcome and sympathise, but also to damage and harm. Just as often we behave indifferently to others' experience or – taken up by our daily routine – we do not even realise what others are experiencing. Nevertheless, we are in the area of "normality" when none of these modalities is exclusive or dominant.

At this point, however, the difference between the capacity to accept the feeling of others and the capacity – which is different both from a phenomenological level and on a conceptual level – to share, to care about or feel responsible for others' experience is evident. The latter is the level of sympathising or of fellow-feeling (*mit-fühlen*), which like the previous level, on which it is founded, presupposes the capacity to recognize the experience of others as being different from one's own (that is, to relive the experience of others after it has been experienced by the other: *nach-fühlen*); but it is different because it implies the intention to receive the feeling of the other adequately and to sympathize with it. It is one thing, in fact, to identify with others' experience, and another to recognize it and differentiate it from our own; and yet another to "respond" or "correspond" adequately with the feeling of the other. These are different experiences but connected by a kind of hierarchy: I cannot correspond to and sympathize with your experience if I am not able to identify it as being yours; I am unable to identify and understand it if I am unable to feel it.

In this perspective, all those theories of empathy which do not differentiate experiences profoundly different from each other such as unipathy, empathy and sympathy are far from convincing. Although they are, in fact, connected and stratified phenomena regulated by the same laws, recognizing their characteristics and differences enables us to avoid simplifications and misunderstandings. The term 'empathy' is often associated with 'altruism', 'cooperation' or with the word 'ethics'. A close correlation between lack of empathy and cruelty has recently been proposed. In this research, based among other things on neurological investigations, empathy is defined as "*our ability to identify what someone else is thinking or feeling and to respond to their thoughts and feelings with an appropriate emotion*" (Baron-Cohen 2011: 16). The point is whether it is possible to use the same term to refer to the capacity to feel what another feels *and* to the capacity – as we have diametrically opposite argued – to respond in an emotionally and ethically adequate way to that feeling. In the theoretical perspective of Baron-Cohen, borderline subjects, psychopathic and narcissist subjects are similar in that they have a "zero negative" level of empathy. This kind of research should enable us to outline a line of scientific enquiry into the nature of evil. But if it is really true that a lack of empathic capacity make normal relations with others impossible, it is also true that feeling the experience of others does not necessarily mean we are able to accept it. Incapacity to put ourselves in the others' shoes is a defect belonging to a superior level of empathy which assumes separation between myself and others; an incapacity which – more than deafness to other's experience – is probably due to a lack of capacity to separate one's own experience from that of others which, because it is fused with one's own, becomes invasive and unbearable.

As we have argued when we discussed the ideas on phenomenology of the early twentieth century, and in particular those of Max Scheler, cruelty can even be increased by the empathic capacity. Knowing where the others' weaknesses lie enables me to make him suffer more deeply and radically. It is, on the contrary, sympathy which enables us to "respond in an adequate emotional and ethical way" to the other's experience: if I am capable of discriminating between our experiences and putting myself in the other's shoes, I can most probably (although it is unnecessary) sympathize with him. So we are left with one more question: Is Sympathy (or *mit-fühlen*) the basis of ethics?

5. Empathy, Sympathy and Ethics

The capacity to feel together with the other and to accept his experience is relevant to the relation of the ethical dimension in two ways. Firstly, it enables us to say that it is thanks to this capacity that – with reference to the trolley dilemma we described at the beginning of this essay – we would not find it easy to throw the fat man off the bridge in order to stop the trolley careering down on the five workers. More in general, the closeness of the bodily or relational and psychical tends to make us bring the other close to ourselves and to act in consequence. It is this closeness, based on the sharing of the other's experience, which can generate a sympathetic attitude to experiences which have nothing to do with ethical behaviour. The fellow-feeling (*mit-fühlen*), Scheler notes, is "blind to value", that is, "It's certainly *not* moral to sympathize with someone's pleasure in evil, his chagrin in contemplating goodness or with his hatred, malice or spite" (Scheler 2008: 1). The closeness and affinity which make the other 'like me' open the door, in this way, to another series of moral problems. It is quite easy to sympathize with someone to whom we feel we are similar, a friend, a neighbor; but the question becomes decidedly more complex when we find ourselves up against a diversity which irritates us, which annoys us or creates problems. Empathy is naturally present in relations inside the group: not only a group of friends or a family group, but also a group of bullies who torment their schoolmates or a clan which practices blackmail and the mafia-like control of an area. The real point, then, is to wonder why empathy is not active towards a weaker schoolmate or fellow citizen.

Recognizing that another person – who I feel to be distant, hostile, different or "disgusting" (Nussbaum 2010) – is our "similar" is a process that seems not to be exclusive to our capacity for empathy. Feeling his experience might generate fear, hatred and disgust: basically, a desire to distance ourselves both physically and psychically. Only by appealing to the rational and cognitive sphere can we recognize the other – and not only a friend or whoever we might recognize as being our neighbor – as the owner of objectives, ambitions, hopes and plans – in a nutshell, as a human being – *similar* to me. Cognitive convergence and the recognition of the other as being similar allow us to "put ourselves in the other's shoes" in a way that makes it possible to change our point of view (or that of the group to which we belong or of our social context). This is a further level of empathy (other than unipathy, empathy and sympathy) which can be called "empathizing and cognitive"; an empathy which emerges from logical thinking and which enables us, even in the case of the distant other, to start from the cognitive *recognition* of its being the bearer of properties (Kant 2002) associated to a *knowledge* of its condition, and to make an effort of the imagination to acquire his point of view. The place or the relevance that a moral enquiry might have in this last level of empathy is not a question for this essay. However, it appears evident that reflection, on the relation between morals and empathy cannot exclude an anthropological enquiry which reveals and does not conceal the complexity of the human being, with his most distant origins as the starting-point. Without forgetting, as Musil has said, that man is capable of as much *Critic of pure reason* as cannibalism.

Notes

1   Apart from the obvious reference to Nietzsche (2002), it is Kant who in his *Groundwork for the Metaphysics of Morals* recognizes the difficulty of investigating the intentions motivating the subject to action. The concept of "masking" which "love of the self" tends to create in order to prevent us from examining authentic motives expresses full awareness of the lack of the subject's self-transparency (see Kant 2002: 23).

2   The subject of love is central in Scheler's thinking; he considers it greatly significant in ethics, differentiating it from acts of co-feeling. It is a concept which falls outside the present work focusing on empathic behavior, and the reader is referred to Scheler (especially 2008: 136–206), and the posthumous manuscript *Ordo amoris* (Scheler 1916), written between 1914 and 1916.

Bibliography

Baron-Cohen, S., Leslie, A. M., Frith U. 1985: Does the Autistic Child Have a "Theory of Mind"? *Cognition* 21(1), 37–46.

Baron-Cohen, S. 2011: *The Science of Evil. On Empathy and the Origins of Cruelty*. New York 2011: Basic Books.

Bergson, H. 1944: *Creative Evolution*, trans. A. Mitchell. New York: Random House.

Bettelheim, B. 1989: *The Uses of Enchantment. The Meaning and Importance of Fairy Tales*. New York: Vintage Books.

Boella, L. 2010: Rileggere il Sympathiebuch. In M. Scheler, *Essenza e forme della simpatia*, trans. L. Boella. Milano: FrancoAngeli, 7–28.

Boella, L. 2011: La morale e la natura. In A. Lavazza and G. Sartori (eds), *Neuroetica*. Bologna: il Mulino, 85–107.

Cusinato, G. 2012: Unipatia ed espressività nel «Sympathiebuch» di Max Scheler. In G. Cusinato, R. De Monticelli, M. Schlossberger, Discussione di Essenza e forme della Simpatia. *Iride* (XXV) 65, 153–162.

Damasio, A. R. 1995: *Descartes' Error. Emotion, Reason and the Human Brain*. New York: Avon.

Edmonds, D. 2013: *Would You Kill the Fat Man? The Trolley Problem and What Your Answer Tells Us about Right and Wrong*. Princeton and Oxford: Princeton University Press.

Foot, Ph. 1967: The Problem of Abortion and the Doctrine of the Double Effect. *Oxford Review* 5, 1–7.

Freud, S. 1990: *Group Psychology and the Analysis of the Ego*, trans. J. Strachey. New York/London: Norton & Company.

Frobenius, L. 1921: *Paideuma. Umrisse einer Kultur- und Seelenlehre*. München: Beck.

Gallagher, S., and Zahavi, D. 2008: *The Phenomenological Mind. An Introduction to Philosophy of Mind and Cognitive Science*. London/New York: Routledge.

Gallese, V. 2006: La molteplicità condivisa. Dai neuroni mirror all'intersoggettività. In V. Gallese *et al.* (eds), *Autismo. L'umanità nascosta.* Torino: Einaudi, 207–270.

Geiger, M. 1911: Über das Wesen und Bedeutung der Einfühlung. In F. Schumann (ed.), *Bericht über den IV. Kongress für experimentelle Psychologie in Innsbruck vom 19. bis 22. April* 1910. Leipzig: Barth, 29–73.

Gibson, J. J. 1986: *The Ecological Approach to Visual Perception.* Hillsdale/London: Erlbaum.

Gopnik, A. and Meltzoff, A. N. 1997: *Words, Thoughts, and Theories.* Cambridge (MA): MIT Press.

Greene, J. 2001: An fMRI Investigation of Emotional Engagement in Moral Judgment. *Science* 293 (5537), 2105–2108.

Greene, J. *et al.* 2004: The Neural Bases of Cognitive Conflict and Control in Moral Judgment. *Neuron* 44 (2), 389–400.

Greene, J. 2009: Dual-process morality and the personal/impersonal distinction: A reply to McGuire, Langdon,Coltheart, and Mackenzie. *Journal of Experimental Social Psychology* 45 (3), 581–584.

Haidt, J. 2003: The Moral Emotions. In R. Davidson, K. R. Scherer, H. H. Goldsmith (eds), *Handbook of Affective Sciences.* New York: Oxford University Press, 852–870.

Harris, P. L. 2000: *The Work of the Imagination.* Oxford: Blackwell.

Hartmann, E., von 1869: *Philosophie des Unbewußten. Versuch einer Weltanschauung.* Berlin: Duncker.

Husserl, E. 1989: *Ideas Pertaining to a Pure Phenomenology and to a Phenomenological Philosophy. Second Book: Studies in Phenomenology of the Constitution,* trans. R. Rojcewicz and A. Schuwer. Dodrecht/Boston/London: Kluwer.

Husserl, E. 1977: *Cartesian Meditations: An introduction to Phenomenology,* trans. D. Cairns. Dordrecht: Martinus Nijhoff.

Jaynes, J. 2000: *The Origin of Consciousness in the Breakdown of the Bicameral Mind.* Boston/New York: Mariner.

Kant, I. 2002: *Groundwork for the Metaphysics of Morals,* trans. A. W. Wood. New Haven and London: Yale University Press.

Kohlberg, L., Turiel, E. 1971: Moral Development and Moral Education. In G. S. Lesser (ed.), *Psychology and Educational Practice.* London: Scott Foresman, 410–465.

Lévy-Bruhl, L. 1921: *Primitive Mentality,* trans. L. A. Clare. London/New York: Allen & Unwin/The Macmillan company.

Lipps, Th. 1906, Einfühlung und ästhetischer Genuß. *Zukunft* 54, 100–114.

Masullo, P. 2013, Laddove si dà qualcosa che sente, s'insinua la probabilità di un significato. In M.T. Catena, A. Donise (eds.), *Sentire e pensare. Tra Kant e Husserl,* Milano: Mimesis

Musil, R. 1922: Helpless Europe. A Digressive Journey. In *Precision and Soul. Essays and Addresses,* trans. B. Pike and D. S. Luft. Chicago: The University of Chicago Press 1990, 116–133.

Nietzsche, F. 2008: *On the Genealogy of Morality,* trans. K. Ansell-Pearson. Cambridge: Cambridge University Press.

Nussbaum, M. C. 2010: *From Disgust to Humanity. Sexual Orientation and Constitutional Law*. Oxford/New York: Oxford University Press.

Österreich, T. K. 1910: Die P*hänomenologie des Ich in ihren Grundproblemen*. Leipzig: Barth.

Scheler, M. 1912: The Idols of Self-Knowledge. In *Selected Philosophical Essays*, trans. D. Lachterman. Evanston: Northwestern University Press 1973, 3–97.

Scheler, M. 1916: *Ordo Amoris*. In *Selected Philosophical Essays*, 98–135.

Scheler, M. 2008: *The Nature of Sympathy*, trans. P. Heath. New Brunswick/London: Transaction.

Schilder, P. 1922: *Über das Wesen der Hypnose*. Berlin/Heidelberg: Springer.

Stein, E. 1964: *On the Problem of Empathy*, trans. W. Stein. Dodrecht: Springer.

Stern, P. 1897: *Einfühlung und Assoziation in der neueren Aesthetik. Ein Beitrag zur psychologischen Analyse der ästhetischen Anschauung*. Hamburg-Leipzig: Voss.

Titchener, E. B. 1909: *Experimental Psychology of the Thought Process*. New York: Macmillian.

Thompson, J. J. 1976: Killing, Letting Die, and the Trolley Problem. *The Monist 59*, 204–217.

Volkelt, J. 1876: *Der Symbol-Begriff in der neuesten Aesthetik*. Jena: Dufft.

Wagner S. 2014: Quell' "oscuro ambito di confine e di passaggio tra natura e spirito": sulle tracce dell'empatia dall'estetica romantica a Karl Jaspers. *Studi Jaspersiani* 2, 383–402.

Unowned: First Notes for a Desubjectivised Aesthetics

DARIO GIUGLIANO

> A very human familiarity exists between the tool and the hand.
> H. Focillon, *In Praise of Hands* in *The Life of Form in Art*

> There's still time for me to write all that down and talk about it. But there will come a time when my hand will be far from me and when I then tell it to write, it will write words that are not mine. The time of that other interpretation will dawn and not one word will be left standing on another and every meaning will dissolve like clouds and descend like rain.
> R.M. Rilke, *The Notebooks of Malte Laurids Brigge*

1.

Between the end of the sixties and the beginning of the seventies of the last century, the artist Rebecca Horn produced a series of works whose main theme was the possibility of having an extension of the human body, in particular of the limbs or upper parts. The first of these works that come to mind at the moment, and which are useful for my introduction and for later discussion of the topic I wish to discuss in this essay, are three works of the period 1968–1972 whose titles in English (the language which has invaded, and continues to invade, all the cultural production of Europe and the world since the second half of the twentieth century) are: *Arm Extensions* (1968), *Finger Gloves* (1972) and *Pencil Mask* (1972). I remember them well as being three works typical of the artistic production of the so-called neo avant-garde of the second half of the twentieth century, the poetics of collective subject which, connected ideally with the dictates of the so-called historical avant-garde, drew inspiration, as it were, from its aesthetic rest, and removed from the political, social and economic, or overall cultural, events following the two world wars, brought back basic ideas and movements. I shall summarize them here in order to approach what will be the conclusion of the essay, taking for granted that all three of the works have a theme in common.

First, however, we need to make clear that what will be described here will be a kind of base note a precipitate (to be considered as such) of something much more complex which will question the state of western art (and not only art) as it was becoming in the recent centuries of the so-called modern age. What is being questioned here is the form of representation; so, in a way, we can consider the object of my description as a "partial object" (in the kleinian psychoanalytic sense) of the overall artistic character of Rebecca Horn, whose works are presented in a more complex way bringing into play so-called performance art. But so far this is a superficial description of the works.

The first, *Arm Extensions*, is the naked body of a woman with her back to us, whose upper limbs, from halfway up the arms down as far as the floor, are covered by two large cylindrical wrappings of red padded fabric. The lower part of the bust, from the height of the false ribs down to the ankles, is criss-crossed with bandages made of the same fabric and of the same colour.

The second, *Finger Gloves*, whose title, as for the other two works, illustrates the artifact that is about to be put on, worn on a specific part of the body (arms and trunk, hands, head), shows a woman (the same one) putting on special gloves with long linear attachments which materially elongate the fingers of the hand.

The third, *Pencil Mask*, is a mask covering the whole head of the woman, made of strips of cloth which cross over each other to form rectangles, with pencils in the intersections.

As we have said, this description does not do justice to the complexity of the whole work of art. In fact, it is something which goes far beyond the mere production and exhibition of an artifact, as indeed, on the one hand, all western art from its origins, has led us to think and expect from an artist and his work, and on the other all so-called avant-garde art from the early decades of the twentieth century to the present. We know full well that from futurism on, the status of works of art has changed radically, opening itself out to aesthetics and in such a way that the work tends more and more to lose its aim of representation and its static nature (as an artifact, in fact), so that it begins to assume an 'open' condition, in progress, 'performative'. Almost as if that typically romantic tension, which tended to merge different artistic expressions into a single whole (the Wagnerian *Gesamtkunstwerk*), a synergy of the arts of time (music, dance, theatre) were extended to every form of art (the special and/or visual arts). It is by no means by chance, in line with this, that gradually there emerged the dominant aesthetic theories of modernity, with their focus on the moment of doing, of creating, producing becoming central. In art, therefore, it is recognized that the main thing is the character of activity and what counts in the basic identification of the artistic act is its poietic, creative nature: the real nature of art is in the doing, in the process which leads to the artifact which, as such, is to be considered as a mere accident whose only function is in allowing the so-called enjoyer (a basic key term)[1] to undertake a journey back to the origin of the creative process. The artifact, then, according to this conception of art, is only a means of (attempting) getting into contact with a process in which the whole creative *act* takes place, and by going over this process we can try to arrive at that initial germinal cell which was the origin of the whole.

The problem with a great deal of contemporary art is that of getting beyond the artifact, in a certain sense. What ends up by being exhibited is not, therefore, the real aim of the entire artistic effort, which, on the contrary, is something which is much more complex of which the artifact simply plays a part. This something, in its turn, is not a referent, the ideal meaning which the sensible signifier, represented by the work, points to; it coincides, rather, with the whole act of performance in its complex development. Seen from this perspective, the works of Horn we have described take on a value which we could say is documentary or commemorative, aiming to give us a certain testimony of the act of performance within which, apart from anything else, the artifact itself functions as an *instrumentum dicatum*.

From a banal referential point of view, however, we can understand these works as being an indication of the extensive-prosthetic character of so-called instrumental appendages which, in our present-day information society, have evolved towards a dematerialization of so-called technological support. This, of course, as we have already suggested, is a flat, superficial interpretation, but nevertheless we shall always need to consider its basic irreducibility as is proper to any preliminary in a hermeneutical comparison. What remains for us to ask is something about its critical character – it does not matter here whether it is manifested or not, whether aware of it or not – about this fact which, by its very nature, would end up by taking on the character of a condemnation. Would these works not be illustrating the future of the human in an era in which sensibility risks being constantly numbed by technique – an era which it seems has lasted for thousands of years, but which in the last century has undergone exponential growth?

Basically, it is as if we were able to take in all the precarious sense of a more or less total submission by the so-called human sphere of sensibility to what is evidently a medium that could only be technical-technological and the same condition of 'extension', which is conceptually explicitly present in the same way as at least one of Horn's works is able to testify to immediately. Here we have a key term: immediacy. There is nothing in the technical paradigm that could ever be immediate, since everything has to pass through the technical medium. This, in fact, is true of every thought of the technical or technological kind as such, as a rational discourse which begins with and with a view to the technical: that it cannot exclude the use of this in the medium term, with which the subject is able to relate to the world. Therefore, there can never be a technique which operates without some kind of media, able to set up a relationship, which would otherwise be impossible, between the subject and the world, in fact it would be better to say, above all, when the media coincides with parts and mechanisms, also derivable by straightforward conceptual precision, of the subject. This is so, for example, with so-called techniques of the body which in the late stage of the modern age Marcel Mauss reflected upon for the first time. Actions related to an idea of bodily immediacy which are apparently spontaneous, such as spitting and blowing your nose, are really the outcome of complex practices whose acquisition and use in time, such as the application of a set of procedures, makes them able to be experienced, once interiorized, according to their natural emergence from their so-called bodily manifestation.

And yet, what seems to be happening in the models of life being propagated everywhere, from the advertising of information multinationals to the more or less dystopic forecasts of so many publications, the possible forms (from the traditional literary form to the more or less recent forms of the moving image from the cinema to video art) seem to be taking on more and more often the (optimistic) semblance of a promise, an expectation of immediacy which totally eliminates all barriers between the self and the world, between the self and others, a guarantee of total universal connection. It is starting from this kind of expectation which is, in fact, a promise, that increasingly models itself on a plan which is that of economic-financial global capital, which recent theories such as those of a "covive intelligence" (Lévy 1999) – which has as its basis the old Aristotelian idea of the relation between potency and act – and that of a "connected intelligence" (de Kerckhove 1997), in some way connected with the previous one, even if much less brilliant in his involuntary bold attempt to understand what one might describe as a general human condition, both the cause and the effect of the pervasive technological flood as the formation of an increasingly more sensibly definable – at least on the level of its purely numerical calculation – "noosphere", according to Teilhard de Chardin (1959). If, as suggested by the Stagirite in *De Anima*, there is a correspondence between the soul and the hand (Aristotle 1991: 57–58), the tool (*organon*) par excellence according to ideas from Anaxagoras to Heidegger, through the school of Averroes, Scholasticism, the Renaissance tradition from Pico to Bruno, a tool which as such is empty or capable of assuming indefinite forms, we cannot avoid ascertaining the character of this conceptual genealogy which, according to a felicitous phrase of Leroi-Gourhan's, assigns the hand to subjection to language and so to the double register of two practices related to the phonetic apparatus (the mouth) and the activity of writing (and of making signs in general).

Basically, the act of signing, of leaving signs, has always indicated a more general practice related to engraving, just as this relates to the possibility of leaving a mnestic trace, the basis of all historiography, as the accumulation and management of documental traces. This is what has linked, from the beginning the skill of writing as a way of controlling objects (management control, in fact, the archive-registry of assets) to the condition of a violence which is managed, moderated and consequently deferred.[2]

2.

On 19 November 1971, the American artist Chris Burden, during a performance entitled *Shoot*, at the F-space Gallery in Santa Ana, California, had an assistant (a friend) shoot him in the left arm with a rifle. The performance, which we can see in a video made at the time, was no other than an action which wounded the artist, who had planned it in every detail. It was he who, in an interview published in the magazine *High Performance* (Moisan 1979), said that he was not particularly interested, in this as in other later actions, in the violence of the action itself – an aspect which is present but not prevalent in Burden's artistic actions,[3] at least on the level of immediate evidence, as in a basic reflection of the relationship between a temporal risk as a condition of the subject's total exposure to the event's taking place and the possibility of a programmed organization of the articulation of moments of life in time. In this sense, the violence of the moment shows explosively the friction between the plan, as a possible programming and absolute control, and exposure to the ungovernable risk of events taking place: it is planned, therefore, that at a certain time on a certain day, in a precise place, you will be hit in the left arm by a bullet from a .22 long rifle. If we consider this performance of Burden's in a longer time perspective, we can place it at the end of a period of evolution, which sees in the possibility of the creation of a certain temporal image the condition of a certain emancipation of the human species as a whole. The image of time that this refers to is clearly that which is conveyed by the mechanism of clocks. From an analogical point of view, these, apart from symbolizing how much time the sun, in a gravitational system of the Ptolemaic kind, takes to run its course, from its reflection within so-called human perception, merge in a spatial synthesis the two moments of the motion, rectilinear and circular, which are usually considered to be opposites. In reality – and it is this fundamental type of representation of time which clearly indicates it – the circle must always be seen as the development of a line which turns on itself. Time and space, therefore, are interconnected at the representative level of their mechanical and geometrical organization. It is from this that the idea of organization and control of a temporal dynamic derives, the representation of which reduces the image to an articulation of mechanical elements that move in synchrony with each other, and the step is not only short, but absolutely immediate. Conversely, this mechanization of temporal dynamics finds its mirror-correspondence in the basic condition of so-called exteriorization. If there is, in fact, something which characterizes the human, this might be found in this basic condition of bringing out, from language to all that relates to the possibility of modification of the environment in interacting with itself, from movement organized in technical matters, in that every being amounts to itself alone as the foundation of its living structure.

What is important, therefore, is not so much to consider the possibility of finding a way of measuring the temporal dimension as to evaluate that technical process which submits that dimension to an exteriorizing mechanization. And indeed, never could there be such as a way of measuring if not with a technical process, as a last resort technological, thanks to that dimension of exteriorization in a device of a technical kind, as a self-aware condition of expression, so typically human. Now – and this is a basic point – it is not always that a self-aware expression ends up by completely and definitively expressing the human as such. And indeed, at the very moment the temporal dimension is exteriorized, objectifying it in a mechanical-type representation, we are already clearly using a technical paradigm as an autonomous system compared to the human which not only brings it into being, but which is its only basic justification of the temporal dimension itself. Who, if not man, could ever be aware of time as change? Who else could have awareness of this change which is time?[4] It is an awareness that clearly cannot pass exclusively for a mechanical-type representation.

Going back to the reflections of Leroi-Gourhan, we might consider the relation that is established, historically, between this way of mechanical representation of time to be the overall condition of this as an exteriorization and organization which is more and more systemic of the technical paradigm, as the basis of an evolution of the human species into forms which at first glance might seem paradoxically only regressive. After all, the example of Burden's performance suggests the existence of the necessity, by now well-defined, of a management of the time dimension which is totally mechanized in the possibility of representation which can completely disregard, by virtue of this mechanized representation, its evenemential dimension. This desire for the possibility of control and management of the temporal dimension with reference to the subject, which is no more than the desire for control and management of the human, not to say (literally) animal or generically-speaking living dimension of the subject, in that it is subject to time, is both the cause and the effect of a mutation of reduction of the human-animal-living being to a machine or an organized organic set which can be dealt with numerically, therefore organized on the basis of the possibility of repetition, which can be calculated. But it is not so much a reduction of man to a computable automaton that we have here, as much as the possibility of a double level from which to redefine epochal representation which consists, on the one hand, of a regression of man towards inferior biological forms, and on the other, an exteriorization of characteristics which until now have been considered typically human, such as the management of rational thinking. This latter aspect, of course, is part of a process which began relatively recently with the invention of the automobile and the steam engine. And it was the harnessing of steam which was to permit the "exteriorization of muscle power" (Leroi-Gourhan 1993: 246), at the beginning of this evolutionary-regressive process in progress, which while, on the one hand, as Leroi-Gourhan points out, was to bring about "the hand separated from motor function" (Leroi-Gourhan 1993: 245–249), and on the other, was not able, at the same time as it began to enjoy freedom, to give to this member of the body a simple function of vigilance over the machine, not to end up in a general dulling of sensibility or aesthetic dimension.

And here we are back to the starting point.

In fact, if we should wish to find a point of contact between these two artistic sensibilities, so different from each other, and for which we used the 'artistic' examples of Rebecca Horn and Chris Burden, we could certainly find it in the basic spirit which unites both, theirs as well as those of a great many more contemporary artists. There are, in fact, many artists whose works, explicitly or not, contribute to the warning: the inexorable dulling of sensibility which, with time, will cancel itself out – and this at a moment in history when everything seems to point to an incitement to enjoyment but which will be more and more restricted to the sphere of idiotism-onanism-privatization. It is no accident that recent surveys report that twenty percent of websites offer pornographic material. It is this voyeuristic matter to which we must now give our attention. In order to do it, we can be guided by the reflections of a great writer. But first it would be better to 'dig' into the meaning and associations of a word.

3.

Pornography is a compound term deriving from ancient Greek. The first of the two words of which it is made up inevitably draws our attention immediately. In ancient Greek, *porne* means 'prostitute' and *porneia* 'prostitution'; in the *Septuaginta*, the Greek translation of the Old Testament made in Alexandria between the second and the first century BC, the noun *porneia* and the verb *porneuo* are both a metaphorical synonym of 'idolatry', a huge subject which we have no space here to discuss and which we shall leave in the background (for example, Hos 4: 10, 13, 18; Ps 72: 27; Ezek 6: 9). In turn, the word *porne* derives from *pernemi*, which means 'bring to the sale'. Émile Benveniste reminds us that in ancient Greek the verbs indicating the practice of selling are organized on the basis of an opposition.

> "[...] *pōleîn* (πωλειν) 'sell' and also a verb from the root **per-* represented by the present tenses *pérnēmi* (περνηι) and *pipráskō* (πιπρασκω) (aorist *epérasa*, επερασα). Now it is possible to draw a distinction between the two verbs which, at the same epoch, seemed to have been employed concurrently without any difference as to sense. The meaning of the second group can be accurately deduced thanks to its derivation from the root **per-*; this appears also in the adverb *péran* 'beyond', 'on the other side', so that the verb will have meant 'to cause to pass, to transfer'. Thus originally the group of pérnèmi did not evoke the idea of a commercial transaction, but the act of transferring. It may

have been the ancient custom among these people to transfer from one point to another, or in the market-place, what they wanted to sell: thus *epérasa*, with a personal name as object, signifies 'transfer' or, as we say, 'export' (cf. Il. 24, 752, where the connection between *pérnēmi* and *péran* is clear).

The frequent sense 'to sell' must be considered as secondary: it is the result of a semantic restriction of the root **per-* (Benveniste 1973, book I, chapter ten).

Even more interesting, in my view, is what Benveniste writes a little later, again in relation to this opposition, about the two terms for 'sell': "*pōleîn* 'put a price on, seek a profit' and *pipráskō* or *pérnēmi* 'to sell by transferring the object (at the market)', generally overseas" (Benveniste 1973, *ibid.*). In particular, this sale by transfer is not directly related to goods, such as foodstuffs or commodities in general, but to rather special commodities: human beings.

> "The first uses were concerned with the purchase of slaves or those destined to become slaves. Symmetrically *peráō*, *pipráskō*, etc. 'sell', strictly meaning 'transfer', is applied to prisoners, to captives. Actual commodities, apart from precious materials, were doubtless not involved in this kind of trafficking and were not subjected to the same procedures of purchase and sale". (Benveniste 1973, ibid.)

Giovanni Semerano (2007: 228–229), with his always stimulating Semitic interpretations, points out how these ancient Greek words, in the Akkadian *eperu*, meaning 'pass beyond, go beyond, on the other shore', have a real calque.

What this amounts to is that at the basis of the term indicating the practice of prostitution there is, even before the concept referring to the universal custom of selling and buying, an underlying idea of transport as communication. There is, that is, from its very origin (together with all that such a complicated and intractable expression is capable of conveying even and above all in contrast with its opposite), that which allows a word to contain a meaning referring to the universal custom of selling, along with the metaphorical meaning of communication as transport, and even that of the exploitation and trading of the human body, that of others and one's own. Basically, and in a certain measure, these three universes of meaning inter-communicate, and the borderline, *peras*, also ancient Greek, between one and the other is always difficult to trace and/or identify. The question is one of identification.

4.

We now come to the ideas of one of the greats of English literature. In the early pages of his essay written in response to accusations of the pornographic obscenity of his exhibition of paintings at the Warren Galleries in London, David Herbert Lawrence focuses on the classical opposition of the dialectic relationship between public and private. Lawrence relates this opposition especially to language, which is of course what makes up the objective basis on which every writer insists in analyzing so-called reality. At this level of analysis, the economic metaphors, derived from the world of commerce, abound. One of the poles of contrast is that of a 'majority' which is immediately described as a 'mob' (Lawrence 1929: 236) which "knows all about obscenity" and which, from time to time, takes on the appearance of "mob-meaning", of "mob-reaction", "mob-acquiescence", "mob-indignation", "mob-condemnation", "mob-habit" (Lawrence 1929: 237–239), and even "mob-self", which is up against an "individual self", "For every man has a mob self and an individual self, in varying proportions. Some men are almost all mob-self, incapable of imaginative individual responses. The worst specimens of mob-self are usually to be found in the professions, lawyers, professors, clergymen and so on" (Lawrence 1929: 238). So that all those who have some kind of relationship with production and consequently a privileged acquaintance with the value of truth, as inter-subjective proof and verification modulated on the basis of a shared and stable standard, in Lawrence's eyes represent that which, in a more or less compact way, is in contrast with the incalculability of how much ground is being lost, both indeterminately and excessively, by subjective poetic individuality. "Business – Lawrence adds – is discovering the individual, dynamic meaning of words, and poetry is losing it" (Lawrence 1929: 238). Here we have yet another economic metaphor, and also two economic models which, as they play their game of opposites as well as possible, reflect each other so that, as far as we can see, they produce that irreducible surplus which no unproductive action can claim as its own basic brand. It might be said that here we have the reasons for the sense of the necessity for every constitutive horizon which, by definition, being what it is, at first glance is irrelevant/unrevealed – a basic sense which, like everything that is basic, in which meanings stand out, cancels itself out at the moment it appears. "Poetry – writes Lawrence – more and more tends to far-fetch its word-meanings, and this results once again in mob-meanings, which arouse only a mob-reaction in the individual" (Lawrence 1929: 238).

But if poetry, in its singularity of meaning, describes life in its irreducible and joyous immanence, the economic circularity of a significant objectivity depends totally on humiliating collective suffering. Its name is idiocy. Yet another economic metaphor is used to express the description of the body politic as a collective body.[5] This time it is a basic commercial metaphor deriving from that kind of trading which, although its everyday association is a negative one, has in fact, sooner or later, a deeper root meaning: fraud, swindle, deceit.

> "The public, which is feeble-minded like an idiot, will never be able to preserve its individual reactions from the tricks of the exploiter. The public is always exploited and always will be exploited. The methods of exploitation merely vary. Today the public is tickled into laying the golden egg. With imaginative words and individual meanings it is tricked into giving the great goose-cackle of mob-acquiescence." (Lawrence 1929: 238)

This idea of Lawrence has a tone which clearly suggests – although it may not be his intention – a reference to the past, to the Victorian age, which created the attitudes, and the climate of intolerance, which contributed to reactions to Lawrence's work. His analysis sounds as if he is reacting to that moralizing that he is so much against, as when, for example, he examines

> "the individual meaning of the word *bread*: the white, the brown, the corn-pone, the home-made, the smell of bread just out of the oven, the crust, the crumb, the unleavened bread, the shew-bread, the staff of life, sourdough bread, cottage loaves, French bread, Viennese bread, black bread, a yesterday's loaf, rye, Graham, barley, rolls, Bretzeln, Kringeln, scones, damper, matsen . . . there is no end to it all, and the word *bread* will take you to the ends of time and space, and far-off down avenues of memory." (Lawrence 1929: 237)

This inexhaustibility of signifier, which drifts in the memory in so many directions, belongs, in Lawrence's view, to that side of us which is the "individual. The word *bread* will take the individual off on his own journey, and its meaning will be his own meaning, based on his own genuine imaginative reactions" (Lawrence 1929: 237). All this individual tendency to create associations is well-known and consequently, is exploited on the collective side, in dealing with the public in a way which is always trading and commercial communication, which has its outward expression in advertising, *réclame*.[6] This is no accident, Lawrence adds:

"The American advertisers have discovered this, and some of the cunningest American literature is to be found in advertisements of soap-suds, for example. These advertisements are *almost* prose-poems. They give the word soap-suds a bubbly, shiny individual meaning which is very skilfully poetic, would, perhaps, be quite poetic to the mind which could forget that the poetry was bait on a hook." (Lawrence 1929: 237–238)

American advertisers. These new actors whom Lawrence calls to the scene of his analysis allows us briefly to refer to another text. It is a passage in an essay by Castoriadis whose interpretation, according to the author himself, goes way beyond certain tones that might seem, at first glance, romantic moralizing or anachronistic apocalyptic prophesying.

"Now, what also is dying today are the forms themselves, and, perhaps, the inherited categories (genres) of creation. Cannot it legitimately be asked whether the novel form, the framed-painting form, the theatrical-play form are not outliving themselves? Independent of its concrete realization (as framed painting, fresco, etc.), is painting still alive? One should not become too easily irritated by these questions. Epic poetry has been quite dead for centuries, if not millennia. After the Renaissance, has there been great sculpture, with a few recent exceptions (Rodin, Maillol, Archipenko, Giacometti . . .)? The framed painting, like the novel, like the theatrical play, implies totally the society within which it arises. What, for example, is the novel today? From the internal wearing down of language to the crisis of the written word, from the distractions, diversions, and the way the modern individual lives or rather does not live time to the hours spent in front of the television set, does not everything conspire toward the same result? Could someone who spent his childhood and adolescence looking at television forty hours a week read *The Idiot*, or an updated version of *The Idiot*? Could he gain access to novelistic life and time, could he adopt the posture of receptiveness/freedom necessary to allow himself to become absorbed in a great novel while at the same time making something of it for himself?

Perhaps what we have learned to call the *cultural work* itself is also in the process of dying: the enduring 'object', destined in principle to an indefinite, individualizable temporal existence, and assigned by right to an author, to a social setting, to a precise date. There are fewer and fewer works, and more and more products, which, like the other products of the era, have undergone the same change in the determination of their temporality: destined not to endure, but to not endure." (Castoriadis 1979: 308–309)

Programmed obsolescence, imposed on any artifact of the commercial circuit, which is then transformed, closing itself up in its own circle, and in its makeup able to become a product for sale, ends up, not only in contrast to cultural works, but above all by distorting and debasing their very nature, which is essentially, according to Castoriadis, a temporal mode of being. Castoriadis extracts this mode of being from an analysis of so-called popular cultural works, which were characterized by continuation and continuation in the establishing of forms with which the community could identify – above all by adding creatively to the continual definition and construction of these same forms. It is not, then, an absolute case of a passive process, but a continual 'creative becoming', a flow which is collectively self-organized. This has been replaced by a "mass production of consumable, perishable items" (Castoriadis 1979: 311) which act as 'tranquillizers', rather as happens with the most advanced forms of smartphone: real-time interface devices and, as we said earlier, if what every one of us have is time as an opportunity to self-manage an economy of existence, the function of these technological devices is much greater than that of a simple tool able to enhance certain senses. Without mentioning the opportunities for socializing, which is by now almost completely through the new media. The period in which Castoriadis was writing, of course, had not yet seen the advent of the internet and social networks, but his analysis, which starts from the simple observation of that mass medium of advanced societies of the second half of the twentieth century, television, arrives, I feel, at a result which is absolutely valid in understanding the dynamics of today's society. The concept which is at the basis of Castoriadis's reflection is another economic concept: privatization.

> "Fifty million families, each isolated in its home and watching the television set, represent both 'external' socialization pushed to a hitherto unknown degree and the most extreme sort of 'internal' desocialization, privatization." (Castoriadis 1979: 312)

The subject's shutting himself up inside himself, in a dream of becoming something which can do without relationships with others. Maybe, *mutatis mutandis*, we are talking about nothing other than idolatry in terms of moving the man–god relationship to the person–person relationship. To return to Lawrence, an interesting convergence is found between these reflections of Castoriadis's and what Lawrence says about pornography:

> "The whole question of pornography seems to me a question of secrecy. Without secrecy there would be no pornography. But secrecy and modesty are two utterly different things. Secrecy has always an element of fear in it, amounting very often to hate. Modesty is gentle and reserved. Today, modesty is thrown to the winds even in the presence of the grey Home Secretaries. But secrecy is hugged, being a vice in itself. And the attitude of the grey ones is: Dear young ladies, you may abandon all modesty, so long as you hug your dirty little secret." (Lawrence 1929: 243)

Considering the huge investment, also in Western government, geopolitical and transnational technical-economical terms, in questions of privacy and privatization, it might be said that this tendency towards secrecy, as a closing of the presumably self-sufficient subject, always tempted by idealism, might be a way of interpreting this age of ours, above all on the level of perception by the senses, which should, of course, be the field of competence of aesthetics. This interpretative key might open the door of a social hermeneutics to the possibility of a great attempt by the above-mentioned economic-political system to allow the subject to recover, starting from his condition of 'secrecy', which by virtue of the findings of the techno-economic system can only seem to be in all its nature exhilarating. Could any subject, in today's world, ever try to have access to this prospect of secrecy if not a part of the system of consumption of the so-called free market? All possibility of demand, even of the most transgressive kind, would already be provided by the endless range of offers.

5.

We are nearing the conclusions of this essay. We started it by describing works of two artists who, like all contemporary artists, almost always involuntarily work in obedience to the techno-economic system whose generically aesthetic field, of which the artist is part, have given, in the eighteenth and above all the nineteenth centuries, the basis of its structural definition starting from consumption and enjoyment, and contributing in a definitive way to the transformation of capitalism from productive to consumeristic. Both of these artists, each in his own way, expresses a personal cry of suffering, no matter whether consciously or not (in fact, for the aims of this essay, the more this characteristic is unconscious, the clearer the overall confirmation of the character of this age of ours) – a cry of suffering for the inexorable weakening of sensibility – witness to a backward tendency in the evolution of what is human, animal and vital. Returning to the ideas of Leroi-Gourhan, we can say that an evolution of man, as we are in the habit of seeing it, must necessarily go through a period of reduction in and adaptation of its 'organs' and basic makeup of its 'states'.

> "But what those early science fiction writers failed to see is that no change is possible without the loss of the hand, the teeth, and consequendy of erect posture. An anodontic human race living in a prone position and using such forelimbs as it still possesses to push buttons is not completely inconceivable, and in certain works of science fiction we find 'Martians' or 'Venusians' who come close to this evolutive ideal. But have we the right to say that such beings would still qualify as human beings?" (Leroi-Gourhan 1993: 129)

When we deliberately disclaim any interest in questions relating to a definition of the human, we have to take note of the fact that whatever refers to the species to which we belong is undergoing considerable and irreversible transformation. It is a transformation which will be more and more what we are in the habit of recognizing as prone to substantial irrelevance. It most immediate consequence, in the field of aesthetics, will be an effective emptying of meaning of the so-called individual and social function of what in the modern age we see as being artistic practice, which will be more and more seen as the adoption and effect of widespread subjectivity – the subject himself not being "a fixed possession" (Weizsäcker 1968: 173), but more and more obviously the effect of a function of the (cultural) collective kind.

A mankind which, evolving in its entirety, regresses, in terms of its individual elements, to the state of the mollusk, might be a credible future possibility bearing witness to the 'maturation' of the present-day situation where our fellows are going more and more in the direction of an immobile condition of the production of standardized behavior which was considered, until a certain period, damaging to our so-called basic individual dignity. Art, as a (middle-class) dream giving access to a subjective freedom (of the feelings) can only be, as it already is (and has been) the first sacrifice made on the altar of this global project.

Notes

1   As we have seen, the concept of enjoyment (fruition) goes back a long way, to Scholastics (a necessary reference, for example, is the *Books of Sentences* by Peter Lombard and the *Commentary* on these sentences by Thomas Aquinas) and, before this, to Patristics. The common point of departure for scholastic philosophers, in fact, is Augustine who, in his *De doctrina christiana* (book I, 8–9), while describing the difference between use (and abuse) and enjoyment, uses a metaphorical example of the journey, a move from one place to another, as a point of arrival which also represents the longed-for source to which to return: "Quomodo ergo, si essemus peregrini qui beate vivere nisi in patria non possemus, eaque peregrinatione utique miseri et miseriam finire cupientes, in patriam redire vellemus, opus esset vel terrestribus vel marinis vehiculis quibus utendum esset ut ad patriam, qua fruendum erat, pervenire valeremus; quod si amoenitates itineris et ipsa gestatio vehiculorum nos delectaret, conversi ad fruendum his quibus uti debuimus, nollemus cito viam finire et perversa suavitate implicati alienaremur a patria, cuius suavitas faceret beatos: sic in huius mortalitatis vita peregrinantes a Domino, si redire in patriam volumus, ubi beati esse possimus, utendum est hoc mundo, non fruendum, ut invisibilia Dei, per ea quae facta sunt, intellecta conspiciantur, hoc est, ut de corporalibus temporalibusque rebus aeterna et spiritalia capiamus" ("Suppose we were travellers who could live happily only in our homeland, and because our absence made us unhappy we wished to put an end to our misery and return to our homeland: we would need transport by land or sea which we could use to travel to our homeland, the object of our enjoyment. But if we were fascinated by the delights of the journey and the actual travelling, we would be perversely enjoying things that we should be using; and we would be reluctant to finish our journey quickly, being ensnared in the wrong kind of pleasure and estranged from the homeland whose pleasures could make us happy. So in this mortal life we are like travellers away from our Lord: if we wish to return to the homeland where we can be happy we must use this world, not enjoy it, in order to discern 'the invisible attributes of God, which are understood through what has been made' or, in other words, to ascertain what is eternal and spiritual from corporeal and temporal things") (Augustine 1995: 14–17).
    The metaphor of the journey is used by Augustine to show the difference between utilization, as in the use of a particular tool to achieve a just-as-particular end, and enjoyment, which is the reflection and contemplation of an object by a subject, from a certain distance.

2   On the relation set up between the dimension of the promise, that of memory and the practice of engraving, firstly corporeal and then, by transposition, elevated in the practice of writing to the external supports respect to the human body, see the first paragraphs (at least the first 5) of the *Second Essay* of *On the Genealogy of Morality* (Nietzsche 2008: 35–41), which I have attempted to use, in the sense that I refer to it, in Giugliano 2012.

3   On 23 April 1974, for example, Burden had himself crucified on the rear

bonnet of a Volkswagen (type 1, known as the "Bug") in a small garage in Speedway Avenue, Venice, California. The car into neutral, with Burden lying belly-up with his hands nailed to the roof, was pushed into the road and, after two minutes of noisy acceleration, with the engine roaring, pushed back into the garage.

4 For these topics see Masullo 1995.

5 See Lawrence (1929: 243), where Lawrence identifies, in the fact that "never was the pornographic appetite stronger than it is today", "a sign of a diseased condition of the body politic".

6 Note that the meaning of this word, whose literal meaning is 'a call', takes us into the world of the performative, a world which at the same time is properly more distant than language. In his dictionary, Littré describes the entry *réclame* as a neologism referring to that "Petit article inséré à part des annonces, dans le corps d'un journal, et contenant l'éloge d'un livre, d'un objet d'art, de commerce, etc.", and then adds: "Les plus mauvais ouvrages obtiennent des réclames laudatives".

Bibliography

Augustine, 1995: *De Doctrina Christiana (On Christian Teaching)*, trans. R. P. H. Green. Oxford: Oxford University Press.

Aristotle 1991: *On the Soul (De anima)*. In *The Complete Works of Aristotle. Electronic Edition. The Rivisited Oxford Translation Volume One*, trans. J. Barnes. Princeton (New Jersey): Princeton University Press.

Benveniste, E. 1973: *Indo-European Language and Society* (1969), trans. E. Palmer. Miami: University of Miami Press.

Castoriadis, C. 1979: Social Transformation and Cultural Creation. In *Political and Social Writings. Volume 3, 1961–1979: Recommencing the Revolution: From Socialism to the Autonomous Society*, trans. D. A. Curtis. Minneapolis/London: University of Minnesota Press 1993, 300–313.

de Kerckhove, D. 1997: *Connected Intelligence. The Arrival of the Web Society*. Toronto: Somerville House Books.

Giugliano, D. 2012: 'Istoriare il corpo. Sull'incisione storiografica.' *Discipline filosofiche* XXII (1), 171–183.

Lawrence, D. H. 1929: *Pornography and Obscenity*. In *Late Essays and Articles*, James T. Boulton (ed.). Cambridge: Cambridge University Press 2004, 233–253.

Leroi-Gourhan, A. 1993: *Gesture and Speech*, trans. A. Bostock Berger. Cambridge (MA)/London: MIT Press.

Lévy, P. 1999: *Collective Intelligence. Mankind's Emerging World in Cyberspace*, trans. R. Bononno. Cambridge (MA): Helix Books.

Masullo, A. 1995: *Il tempo e la grazia. Per un'etica attiva della salvezza*. Roma: Donzelli.

Moisan, J. 1979: 'Interview with Chris Burden.' *High Performance* 5, 9.

Nietzsche, F. 2008: *On the Genealogy of Morality*, trans. K. Ansell-Pearson. Cambridge: Cambridge University Press.

Semerano, G. 2007: *Le origini della cultura europea*, vol. II (*Dizionari etimo-*

logici. Basi semitiche delle lingue indeuropee) tomo I (*Dizionario della lingua greca*). Firenze: Olschki.

Teilhard de Chardin, P. 1959: *The Phenomenon of Man*, trans. B. Wall. New York: Harper.

Weizsäcker, V. von 1968: *Der Gestaltkreis. Theorie der Einheit von Wahrnehmen und Bewegen*. Stuttgart: Georg Thieme Verlag.

CHAPTER 11

Posthuman Pathicity: The Neoenvironment

AGOSTINO CERA

Non c'è davvero altro che conti che sentirsi l'anima in corpo.
Rocco Scotellaro

This essay will briefly set out the outcome of a research activity lasting several years which culminated in a proposal for a *philosophy of technology in the nominative case* (filosofia della tecnica al nominativo) grounded on the concept of *Neoenvironmentality* (neoambientalità). Given the limits of such an exposition, the essay will cover the main points of the research as they are to be found in the original sources.[2] The inclusion of this proposal in the present book depends on its intrinsic posthuman component. The term 'posthuman' is not used here in its conventional sense, rather it is used for practical working purposes, 'empty' as it were. This emptiness being filled by having it function as a link to a precise anthropological hypothesis. We hope that just from the making explicit of such a posthuman component (in its heterodox sense) of technology as an epochal phenomenon will emerge some critical points regarding the composite constellation of posthumanism (in its orthodox sense). This without pretending to advance solutions or judgments, however. It will be enough to undermine any presumed certainties while sowing some perplexities.

The proposed thesis is that the phenomenon of *neoenvironmentality* – that is, the decisive effect produced by technology in its systemic version – represents a watershed, beyond which a substantial alteration of the 'man-form' is taking shape. As a consequence, from here any attempt to propose an anthropological hypothesis becomes problematic. In a formula: when technology elevate itself to the status of a totality (in terms of a neoenvironment), it marks the limit of the human; and thus an eventual 'man's after', namely a possible posthuman threshold.

Saying that technology marks a real anthropological limit implies the explication of the parameter used to distinguish such a threshold. The position taken here is based on the epochal awareness that the 'essence' of man can no longer be predicated. This awareness, however, does not mean that we must give up identifying some set of elements that can characterise man in a particular way. In this regard, definitions such as 'human essence' or 'human nature' are replaced here by that of *anthropic perimeter*. And since the barycentre of this perimeter is to be attributed to a specific pathos – that is to say, to the specific findingness that attunes man to his corresponding vital space – it is within this pathic horizon that we have to find the posthuman threshold. This is a further justification for including this essay in the present book.

By altering specific human pathicity (*thauma* and *theorein*), technology compromises the stability of the anthropic perimeter towards a post-human condition, which is potentially ferine because it is no longer wordly but (neo)environmental. So: *the posthuman threshold is the basic effectual consequence identified by a philosophy of technology in the nominative case, which finds out the essential character of contemporary technology in its rise to the status of neoenvironment.* That is to say, in its capacity to *erode the anthropic perimeter*.

We shall begin by clarifying the formulas 'philosophy of technology in the nominative case' and 'anthropic perimeter'. This represents a necessary preliminary step in order to interpret technology as *neo-environment*.

Before beginning, it is necessary to give a preliminary reply to an objection that seems reasonable to some extent, but that also proves to be ineffective regarding the real question, which is here at stake. This objection is the following: there is no necessary correspondence between 'animality' – granted that such a thing really exists – and the so-called environmentality. On the contrary. It must be clear that the theoretical proposal advanced here does not state such an equation. In other words, it is in no way claimed that environmentality represents the special way of being of that set of living beings that we conventionally define 'animals'. Even if the hypothesis of animal environmentality turned out to be a simple anthropological projection, what would really matter for our present discourse is the capability of such a projection to establish *ab intra* (i.e., from within the human condition) a criterion of recognisability for man, namely its capability to mark a boundary beyond which human being would fail to recognize itself as such. Therefore, the equation between environmentality and animality, conceived as a thought experiment, works only as a necessary term of comparison to indicate that an 'environmentalized' man – that is, a man inhibited in his worldhood. And this seems to be the human type produced by technology in its systemic version – would be unrecognisable to the man himself.[3]

1. Philosophy of Technology in the Nominative Case

Our clarification of formula 'philosophy of technology in the nominative case' will make reference to the words of Franco Volpi, who inspired it. Volpi writes: "There is a risk: that yet another genitive philosophy will be produced. I mean, a reflection whose only function is ancillary and subordinate [...] the risk of numerous genitive philosophies [...] is to reduce philosophical thought to a noble *anabasis*, to a strategy withdrawn from the great questions to take refuge in problems of detail [...] So one asks oneself: is philosophy of technology in the nominative case (*filosofia della tecnica al nominativo*) possible?" (Volpi 2004: 146–147). In our view, these words require an affirmative response: such a philosophy is possible. The reasons for this response are the following.

(1) Nominative is that philosophy of technology which, by claiming its full autonomy, takes on the responsibility of demonstrating the reality of its object. In fact, according to what Jacques Ellul calls "criticism of nominalism", so-called 'technology' is only a philosophical totem to which "no reality corresponds" (Ellul 1984). On this basis, philosophy of technology in the nominative case defines itself by rejecting all those 'in the genitive case' approaches which debase the philosophical idea of technology by fragmenting it into a plethora of single items (*techniques* or *technologies*), each of which has its own special issues. The structural defect of these approaches lies in inadequate understanding of what still nowadays has to be considered the epigraphs of *technisches Zeitalter*, namely that "the essence of technology is by no means anything technological" (Heidegger 1953: 4). The totally circumspect point of view of the aspiring "technicians of technology" miss the fact that individual technologies are no more than the instruments which instrumentality needs in order to achieve an autotelic rank, i.e. to become an aim in itself. The *philosophy of technology in the nominative case is therefore first and foremost that kind of approach which opts for 'technology' against 'techniques'*, since it recognizes its own object as the actual form of the world and "subject of history" (Anders 2002b: 9, 271–298). Its task is "simply to present, by means of a comprehensive analysis, a concrete and basic interpretation of the technological phenomenon" (Ellul 1964: xxxvi).

(2) However, the philosophy of technology in the nominative case pretends to be neither a system nor a method. It cannot, otherwise it would be reduced within a context which, regardless of its inspiration, would be organic within the technological *ratio* of its effects.[4] Instead, such a philosophy of technology should be defined a *habitus*, a style. It has an innate phenomenological and impressionistic attitude, which trusts in its diagnostic capability but avoids pronouncing epochal judgments. A concrete example of this unsystematic *habitus* is Günther Anders's *"philosophical anthropology in the epoch of technocracy"*, which while claiming an analytical and hermeneutic strictness at the same time intends to remain an *"occasional philosophy"*, i.e. a philosophy, which starting from the consideration of precise experiences and phenomena arrives at a "systematic *après coup*" (Anders 2002b: 9, 10). Which is eventually found to be systematic only afterwards.

On the basis of its 'hodological' option – namely, in its refusal to be put in the cage of a method – the philosophy of technology in the nominative case refers to the experience and example of those who have been shown such a diagnostic talent on the ground. A talent which, in the last resort, corresponds to nothing but an authentic historical sense, a genuine feeling for their own times. Among these 'masters of style' we can count Martin Heidegger, Jacques Ellul, Günther Anders, Ernst and Friedrich Georg Jünger, Arnold Gehlen, Ernst Kapp, Lewis Mumford and Gilbert Simondon.[5] Nevertheless this list does not equate to the building of a pantheon. Despite their value as examples, these authors will be used here functionally in relation to the specific purpose we try to achieve.

(3) Although technology is not an anthropological matter *tout court*, it always involves the question of man. Therefore, the philosophy of technology in the nominative case opts for a conscious *anthropological involvement* and so for the 'neohumanism' of Ellul and Anders, that is to say against the anthropological indifference (only presumed, by the way) of Heidegger. Such an involvement expresses the awareness of the inextricable connection between man and technology. Anthropogenesis and technogenesis are synonyms: behind and within any position regarding technology there is concealed an anthropological and cosmological assumption.[6] Thinking about technology implies *ipso facto* thinking about the world to which it intends to give a form and, at the same time, about those who, while realizing such a form of world, have to place themselves within it.

On the basis of the positional character of its anthropological presupposition (i.e., the anthropic perimeter), the philosophy of technology in the nominative case takes up a position by taking on the task of safeguarding man's need and possibility for his self-recognition. Because the fundamental task of that living being, whose beginning is "in knowing it [i.e., in knowing such a beginning]"[7] is in always wanting (and being able) to know it.

(4) As a consequence of its conscious non-neutrality, the philosophy of technology in the nominative case chooses an *interstitial position*, so removing itself from two complementary temptations. The first, the avoidance of the paradoxical outcome of so-called "engineering" (*ingegnerismo*), namely those approaches characterized by a too much disenchanted rationalism that, while refusing to recognize the epochal meaning of technology, end up by making it an irrefutable *positum* and therefore an *idolum*.[8] The second, the avoidance of that divinatory determinism, which involves even some of the most important attempts to ask philosophical questions about technology.

While recognizing its intrinsic historicity, it is not intended to present the philosophy of technology in the nominative case as a new philosophy of history which is always, at best, a secularized disguise of unfulfilled religious angst.[9] It takes up its diagnostic attitude to the full without pretending to become a historical mantic. The philosophy of technology in the nominative case is constitutively *unzeitgemäß* (untimely) and it is only for this reason never *antiquiert* (obsolescent), only in this way always indispensable in its own time.

2. The Pathos of the Human: The Anthropic Perimeter

2.1 Ek-staticity and Worldhood

Now that we have explained the meaning and function of the philosophy of technology in the nominative case, we can move on to the *anthropic perimeter*, a definition which synthesizes the attempt to propose here and now a plausible response to the philosophical question about man. The anthropic perimeter represents what remains of the human once we set aside a substantialist interpretation; i.e., it is *the possibility of continuing to say something essential about man once we have acknowledged the impossibility of saying what his essence is.*

Therefore this definition has to be considered a fundamental legacy of those philosophical-anthropological considerations that, from Herder to Gehlen, gave birth to the paradigm of *Mängelwesen* (deficient being). Such a paradigm is characterized by a destructive and a constructive side. The former dismisses the substantialist interpretations, producing as its outcome an *anthropology of negativity* expressed in the ratification of that structural deficiency – first of all biological – with which the human being is naturally equipped. This dismissal, however, is affirmatively counterpointed, so it culminates by becoming a new paradigm of relational inspiration in which the deficit (*Mangel*) positioned at the basis of the deficient *imago hominis* acquires a paradoxical, because indeterminate, fullness. The peculiarity of man is not to be found in his 'What' any longer, but in his 'How', i.e. in a fundamental 'disposition'. His authenticity is all about his unique way of 'placing himself'. With the transition from *natura hominis* to *conditio humana*, man's way of being emerges as a constellation. As a perimeter. *Man is characterized on the basis of the relation he establish with the in-which (the where) of his* dasein. In other words: man's being corresponds to the special way in which he *is within (in-sistere)* the framework (*Umgebung*) that surrounds him. Such a 'being-in' (*in-sistere*) is always already a 'being at a distance': such an *in-sistere* always and already corresponds to an *ex-sistere*. Man's Dasein is ek-sistence: this is his fundamental peculiarity. Compared to that of other living beings, man's *position* is *peculiar* in that it is characterized as a *positioning*, since he himself contributes in a decisive way to the building of his own vital space (his *oikos*), so imprinting a specific form on himself, too. We shall call this natural human feature *worldhood*,[10] with explicit reference to Jakob von Uexküll's *Umweltlehre* and the distinction he makes between man and animal, where the former emerges as a 'worldly being' (*Weltwesen*) because he has a world (*Welt*), and the latter as an 'environmental being' (*Umweltwesen*) because he has a mere environment (*Umwelt*).

This hypothesis summarizes the affirmative side of the defective paradigm and turns negative anthropology into a new kind of anthropology which is not only topological, but *positional*.[11] Man finds himself being *naturaliter* obliged to mould the matter of his own setting to make it habitable. Only once that initial setting or *milieu* (*Umgebung*) has been formed, does it become world (*Welt*), i.e. the specific in-which for man's Dasein.[12] It follows that human adaptation is characterized as a meeting halfway between the initial human givenness – his 'deficient' biological endowment – and that of the setting. In agreement with Heidegger, we can say that the essential peculiarity of man is his *"world-forming"* (weltbildend) ability (Heidegger 1995: 274–366). Being *world-forming*, he is a naturally technological being: he has an intrinsic demiurgic vocation which, as said, makes of him the inevitable moulder of a shapeless matter that existed before him.

On the contrary, the ecological niche of the animal is environment: a natural mould to which it corresponds entirely and immediately. By reference to the animal, the environment expresses itself as an absolute selfgivenness: "it is there ready for the animal as the breast is there for the baby [...] The animal does not come to the world, but the world comes to it" (Anders 1935: 65–66). This means that the animal is unable to experience any setting (*Umgebung*), namely that preliminary framework functioning as an indeterminate background to its concrete vital space. And this means that it is precluded from the possibility of experiencing its own environment *as such* (als solches). Therefore, the basic peculiarity of the animal lies in its *environmentality*, in its being "*poor in world*" (weltarm), as Heidegger affirms (Heidegger 1995: 186–267).

Given these premises, the difference between man and animal cannot be ascribed to a strictly biological perspective, but requires a positioning which, if not ontological, is at least ecological. What makes them different is the relation they have with their corresponding *oikos* (vital space). The *Bauplan* (structure plan) of the animal enables it to insert itself immediately into a specific ecological niche, in which it is fully absorbed until it disappears. In the perfect mixture of "*Merkwelt*" (perception world) and "*Wirkwelt*" (effect world), the vital circle of the animal expresses itself in a circuit-like modality.[13] As a whole, the animal and its ecological niche form an inseparable unity, i.e. an individual or even a monad. This means that the animal has no possibility of experiencing either its own *as such* or that of its environment. 'As such', which corresponds to a differential *dynamis*, that is to the ability to perceive the otherness in itself, namely in 'its being in itself and for itself different from me'. As an environmental being (*Umweltwesen*), the animal is denied such an ability and therefore the possibility to grasp, i.e. *release-be* (Seinlassen), the beings: "*The animal as such does not stand within a manifestness of beings. Neither its so-called environment nor the animal itself are manifest as beings*" (Heidegger 1995: 248).[14]

All this also indicates a structural difference of *adaptive performance* between man and animal. *The animal is apt insofar as it is adapted*, its adaptation being *energheiai, in actu*: from the very beginning, it is ready for its *oikos*. On the contrary, *man is apt insofar as he is adaptable*, his adaptation expresses itself *dynamei, in potentia*. In other words: through his technological-demiurgic capability, he is able to fill the initial distance between himself and his own setting, making of it an *oikos*.

To recapitulate: overcoming the essentialistic approach allows the relational paradigm to emerge, and this coagulates in the image of the *Mängelwesen*, which at first seems exclusively negative. The 'non-essence' of man looks like a mere deficiency only within the organic-biological spectrum, while in a wider horizon – that *onto-ecological*[15] of a positional anthropology – it reveals itself to be a fundamental opening to the 'where of his own Dasein'. Such a natural place for man is the world: a vital space which "is not a *datum*, but a *dandum*" (Accarino 1991: 30). As we said, the collocation (*in-sistere*) of man within such an *oikos* equates to a being at a distance *(ex-sistere)*: in the distance of a disclosed (free) opening.[16] In order to live (that is, *ex-sistere*), man cannot get out of moulding his wordly sphere, which means that it is on the basis of this worldhood that he recognizes himself as man. Just as environmentality defines the animal as such, making an *Umweltwesen*, so worldhood defines man as such, so making a *Weltwesen*.

2.2. De-severance and Earthhood

Our next step concerns the 'debiologizing' of the anthropological structure we have described, in order to protect it from that misunderstanding, to which Gehlen's *Elementary Anthropology* fell victim and exposed his paradigm of *deficiency* to the risk of a mis-leadingly *pauperistic* interpretation. To achieve such a result we need, first of all, to substitute a central element in Gehlen's anthropology: the concept of "*relief*" (Entlastung), with that of "*de-severance*" (Ent-fernung).[17] Precisely because of its biologistic, zoocentric origin, the idea of *Entlastung* is potentially misleading. To interpret human action, as Gehlen does, as being relieving, gives a picture of man constructed on the basis of an initial, and neutral, zoological presupposition. Man is here implicitly thought as a 'simple living being' with 'something more', i.e. a mysterious *conatus*, which by the action (the technology) gradually distances him from a hypothetical initial state of nature which is totally identical to the ferine. Such a reconstruction holds up only if we accept its biologistic premise by which every living being is first and foremost an environmental being. This premise is no longer valid if we adopt onto-ecological terms, according to which, to that being recognized as 'man' is attributed a special 'worldly vocation', namely the natural ability/necessity to mould his own setting, so making it an *oikos*/world. This means that the initial condition for the human being is not to be found in its proximity to its own ecological niche, rather, as said, in its distance from it. As a consequence, the basic directionality of his worldforming action is that of de-severance, approximation. In other words: as the passing of the original condition of "world-strangeness" (*Weltfremdheit*) or "world-openness" (*Weltoffenheit*).[18] Action, and technological action, is essentially de-severant, since man is by nature a "creature of distance (*Wesen der Ferne*)" (Heidegger 1929: 135).

Seen in this perspective, the world as such corresponds to the first and fundamental 'de-severed', i.e. the first and essential result of man's de-severant action. Therefore, the world as such embodies the preliminary framework which establishes and orientates the 'within-the-world de-severance', namely the relation between man and other beings.

This point of view brings about a decisive change in evaluating the impact of technology on the present-day life of man, what is usually called *alienation*. Such alienation can no longer be considered a sort of hyper-distancing from our 'natural' *oikos*, as if our state of nature coincides with the identification typical of ferine environmentality. The epochal false movement triggered by technology in its systemic version does not equate to a to the last distancing, rather to a forced approximation, that is a promiscuity. A (con)fusion. It corresponds to the attempt to annihilate the natural preliminary distance between man and world, making them indistinguishable from one another. It tries to fill the cosmological difference between *Welt* (world) and *Menschenwelt* (human world); to eclipse the surplus of *mundus rerum,* reducing it to mere *mundus hominum.*[19] In its systemic version, technology aims at the systematic erosion of our ek-static potential. Such a dynamic, which can be considered the current *telos* of *techne*, represents a fundamental moment in the mechanism of neoenvironmentality which clarifies the real meaning of its 'altering (alienating) effect' on the human condition.

At this point, in order to make the notion of *de-severance* really functional, we need to place it in an appropriate context, freeing the concept of 'world' from its biologistic perspective, namely without restricting it to a physical-biological correlate. Man's authentic ecological niche is made up of elements that are not 'natural', but at the same time necessary: i.e., of all that relates to the so-called 'cultural sphere'. The world has a plurality of dimensions which is precluded to the animal's environment. Therefore, the difference between world and environment is not a simple difference of extension, but a *dimensional difference.* The world corresponds to the establishment of an undivided natural-cultural (physical-spiritual) framework of stabilization for that very special being, who counts among its vital needs the question of making sense. "By the opening of a world, all things gain their lingering and hastening, their distance and proximity, their breadth and their limits" (Heidegger 1936: 23). Like a metronome, the world founds and scans the concrete rhythmic of the human *ex-sistere*. Every specific world that is concretely shaped by man equates to that particular type of framework we call 'epoch'. It follows that the above-mentioned man's worldhood – the *Weltbildung*, i.e. his ability to form worlds – corresponds to his *historicity*, namely the 'non-historical (pre)condition of his making history'. The salient trait of the indissoluble relationship between man and world is the *Geschehen* of *Geschichte*, the historical happening in its authenticity. Therefore, insofar as man is an historical being, he can reveal himself as a worldly and not merely as an environmental being.

Having described the concept of world in a literally 'meta-physical' sense, we need now to make another substitution, this too inspired by Heidegger, indicating as *earth* (Erde) what *Umweltlehre* and Gehlen's anthropology call *Umgebung* (or: setting, *milieu*, objective world). 'Earth' will denotes the *chora*, the worldly-historical *hyle* where the innate demiurgical *dynamis* of man intervenes in order to mould a world every time and so every time let history happen. Given such a premise, the question becomes: "If not a setting or a physical *milieu*, what is the earth?". Preliminarily, we can affirm that it is "the coming-forth-concealing (*Hervorkommend-Bergende*). Earth is that which cannot be forced, that which is effortless and untiring. On and in the earth, historical man founds his dwelling in the world [...] The earth is openly illuminated as itself only where it is apprehended and preserved as the essentially undisclosable, as that which withdraws from every disclosure, in other words, keeps itself constantly closed up" (Heidegger 1936: 24–25).[20] The earth equates to the unmanifested condition for the manifestation of every world. Like Heidegger's *Licthung* (clearing), it scans an aletheiological rhythmic: it reveals itself only by veiling itself, acting as an indeterminate background (*apeiron*) to the appearance of those certainties (*perata*) which are, firstly, the world, and with the world (within it) all the individual beings.

The earth is therefore disclosing, but in itself closed. So, how can its presence be perceived? Does it not risk being reduced to a postulate, the totally outdated re-edition of a hinterwordly hypostasis? But above all, whereas the earth is characterized as being unavailable – otherwise, and eventually, by means of a leap of faith – would it seem, to our eyes, that the world is a world without its background? Without any *Umgebung*? And at that point, how can the world be distinguished from the mere environment? Man from the animal? Again, it is from the dialogue with Heidegger that a possible solution takes shape. With 'earth' Heidegger identifies the *Abgrund* (the 'ungrounded ground') of every world, that which circumscribes it and goes beyond it. It goes beyond it, but without ever transcending it, whenever the sense of total break and separation is attributed to transcendence. The surplus and furtherness of the earth is not of being elsewhere. World and earth are essentially co-present, they belong intimately to each other. What bonds them is that original form of relation which, in citing Heraclitus, Heidegger calls "*Streit*", i.e.

"strife", dispute, *polemos*. "World and earth are essentially different and yet never separated from one another. World is grounded on earth, and earth rises up through world [...] The opposition of world and earth is strife [...] In essential strife, however, the opponents raise each other into the self-assertion (*Selbstbehauptung*) of their essences" (Heidegger 1936: 26). It is obvious that there is a connection between these claims and the well-known Heraclitian fragment (B 53) which celebrates the *polemos* as the most original form of relation: that is, a connection that expresses a fundamental *koinonia*, on the basis of which, and only on this basis, contrasting individualities can achieve a reciprocal emergence and determination. World and earth are not one without the other: what is manifested cannot *be* given without the *Abgrund* that allows it to come into the presence; the producer, in its turn, cannot be given except in concealment, namely in that emptiness that can be revealed as such only in relationship to the fullness produced by the emergence of what is manifested.

Well, if it is true that man is given only insofar as world is given, then the world is given only against the earth as its *Abgrund*. In view of the essential co-belonging of world and earth, worldhood must by implication possess a corresponding *earthhood*. However, the previous question remains unanswered: how can we perceive the earth – or rather, find our own earthhood –, given the fact that the latter is given only within its inextricable strife with the world and given that the *conditio humana* corresponds to a 'being-(always-already)-in-the-world'? Namely, 'in a (specific) world'? The earth can be seen only by contrast: against the background, as *Abgrund* of the emergence of the world. As a consequence, earthhood equates to a movement that is complementary and intrinsic to worldhood. The perception of the earth is at one with perception of the world as such, since the grasp of the world as a whole presupposes a horizon against which it stands out. In this way, we are faced again with the subject of 'as such', of releasing be the beings, i.e. with that differential and relational capacity that establishes the peculiar nature of man in comparison with the other living beings. On the other hand, when we speak of the world we do not refer to a being among others, but to that framework in which man is always already situated – human Dasein is being-in-the-world – even if he is at the same time its 'moulder'. Therefore we can affirm that, in the eyes of its moulder and inhabitant, the world has been always such, without being as such.

So the possibility we have of perceiving the earth lies in and depends on our awareness of the world as such. On releasing it be, or rather fully experiencing that ek-staticity that we have attributed to man as his original peculiarity. But how can such a particular being, which finds himself always already situated in the world, distance himself from it in order to be aware of it as a whole? As can be seen, *earthhood, worldhood and ek-staticity* – to which one must add *historicity*: a kind of synthesis of the other three – are the constituents of a unitary structure, i.e. what in this essay we have called the *anthropic perimeter*. When one of these is missing, the others too are inevitably absent.

To overcome this *impasse* there is a need for a *pathic turn*. Our grasp of the world as such – that is, the aware experience of our own ek-staticity – cannot take a course which is 'active' in the general sense, i.e. logical, gnoseological, practical . . . because these all are *integrally* 'within-the-world picklocks'. On the contrary, such a *passepartout* is to be looked for in the dimension of fully ek-staticity, of pure ex-position: that of *affectio*, pathos. World and earth cannot be either demonstrated or deduced or postulated. World and earth can be only felt.[21]

On the other hand, given the inescapable anthropological precondition of being-in-the-world, the perception of the world as such – namely, the necessary requisite for access to earthhood – must come from inside the world itself, in a 'within-the-world way' and thus *ex post*: i.e., when the world is already made. In his *Fundamental Concepts of Metaphysics*, Heidegger traces the determining factor of the ontological condition of *weltbildend*-man and *weltarm*-animal in the sphere of the *pathemata*, moods (*Stimmungen*). In particular, those basic moods (*Grundstimmungen*) which attune each of them to their respective findingness (*Befindlichkeit*). In the case of the animal/*Umweltwesen*, he finds such an original pathos in *Benommenheit*: that *captivation-enmeshment*, that is the sign of a total integration with one's relative vital space (Heidegger 1995: 236–257). It is an interpenetration which becomes a real fusion and so determines the impossibility of disclosure of any openness. As a result, the animal is consequently unable to access the *as such* of any being, including itself. Its inability to go out of itself depends in this case on its inconsistent self. On this basis, we can say that the animal at the same time has and has not a peculiar findingness. It has it in the sense that *Benommenheit* represents *de facto* the cipher of its ontological condition; it has not it, since its peculiar findingness lies just in the impossibility of feeling it. *Benommenheit* is structurally circular: it falls back on itself, implodes in a monadic outcome. The vital circle of the animal becomes an ecosystemic circuit, so its fundamental pathos essentially corresponds to *apatheia*. Namely, to a sensitivity, which is incapable of self-awareness.

Man/*Weltwesen*, on the contrary, has a totally explicit findingness because his self-awareness achieves a complete evidence. That said, it should not be forgotten that here we are asking such a pathic marker to carry out a very special task: to grasp the *as such* not of a being among others, but of that framework (the world) where man is always already positioned. Moreover, the world as such can only reveal itself *ex post*, and above all exceptionally: as a sort of violation of a 'normal state' marked by a familiarity between man and his ecological niche, which in appearance seems to be not so different from the animal *Benommenheit*. This represents a decisive aspect in understanding the process triggered by technology as an epochal phenomenon. The function of the world as a stabilizing sphere for man's Dasein goes necessarily through an operation of concealment and transfiguration with regard to that open which represents its framework and support. In order to carry out its amniotic function, the 'worldly wrapping' needs to be perceived by the who dwelling in it as a total and untranscendible horizon to which he can release himself completely. It is just this need for stabilization and immunization which generates that pseudo-*Bennomenheit*, i.e., that sort of captivation, which corresponds to the "everydayness" (*Alltäglichkeit*) of "circumspection" (*Umsicht*), that in Heidegger's existential analytic is labeled "inauthenticity" (*Uneigentlichkeit*). In accordance with such a need, the pathos revealer of the world as such must correspond to an exceptional condition, a violation of the everydayness whose special trait is the unhomeliness (*Unheimlichkeit*). The sight of the world as such – namely, the slit which discloses the earth as world's 'ungrounded ground' (*Abgrund*) – is something whose abyssality looks unhomely for the reassuring "reliability" (*Verläßlichkeit*) of worldly-daily-circumspect *amnios*. The pseudo-captivation of circumspect everydayness is the price paid for the stabilization of concrete existence, whereas the clearness of an uninterrupted gaze at the disclosed open (i.e., at the *polemos* between world and earth) would be at the unsustainable cost of a petrifying stasis.

The human need for stabilization/immunization results in a concealment which establishes the within-the-world framework *par excellence*: the everydayness, in the eyes of which the real worldly pathos necessarily looks like a rift, a trauma. This is why Heidegger sees in telluric *Stimmungen* such as "anxiety" (*Angst*) or "boredom" (*Langeweile*) ek-static bridges that shake up the stabilized and captivated everydayness and so lead from the world to the earth. They trigger a *Grundstimmung* which by virtue of its capacity to transcend its own within-the-world rootedness embodies the authentic earthly *pathos*: that which allows the definitive revealing of the 'as such of the world'. For human being, such an exceptional pathic condition corresponds to the full awareness of his own findingness, the maximum self-transparency of his own ex-position. This fundamental mood is the 'wondering horror' of *thauma/thaumazein*, of *theorein/Betrachtung*.[22] The world as such can only be announced by the traumatic way of a "thrust" (*Stoß*), i.e. thrusting the enmeshed reliability of everyday inauthenticity with the unhomely evidence of its bare "that" (*Daß*), with the scandalous gratuitousness of its pure being (Heidegger 1936: 39–40).[23] The everyday enmeshment gives way to the tremors of boredom and anxiety until *thauma* is re-aroused: namely, the pathic rest of that wondering horror which represents the nearest approximation man can achieve to the 'polemic' *koinonia* of world and earth. To the full disclosure of the open. While thrusting his own circumspect and captivated everydayness, man becomes able wholly to assume his own findingness.

The human being is such not only in that he is *weltbildend* (*able to form the world*), but also – to coin a term – *erdfühlend*: *able to feel the earth*.

Insofar as they define the peculiarity of human being compared to every other living being, *ekstaticity, worldhood, earthhood (and historicity)* emerge as *the markers of the anthropic perimeter*. Only in a similar perspective the real significance of technology as a question of philosophy can be entirely understood, because its titanic purpose to become the actual *oikos* for the "creature of distance" equates to the attempt to redesign the anthropic perimeter.

3. The Pathos of the Posthuman: The Neoenvironment

We should now bring together the threads of the argument so far and list the main point of the complex dynamic that leads technology to acquire the status of a neoenvironment. First and foremost, we need a working definition of the term 'technology'. While it can generally be labeled as 'instrumental actions', it takes on a more special character when it aspires to become the *oikos* for present-day humanity. In this sense, 'technology' does not indicate here the totality of single technologies, rather it outlines the worldview that has made them possible and that manifests itself as a very particular historical circumstance: a compound of *disenchantment* (Entzauberung) and *rationalization* (Rationalisierung), under the imperative of *realization* (Realisierung) in terms of *makeability* (Machbarkeit) (Cera 2007: 98–101).

Jacques Ellul provides an incisive summary of this process. Starting from the assumption that "there is no common denominator between the technique of today and that of yesterday" (Ellul 1964: 146), Ellul distinguishes between *technical operation, technical phenomenon and technical system.* "The technical operation includes every operation carried out in accordance with a certain method in order to attain a particular end" (1964: 19). The "technical phenomenon" stands out from the background of technical operations and introduces the technological *ratio operandi* in any human context, that is, it represents "the main preoccupation of our time [...] in every field men seek to find the most efficient method" (1964: 21). The combination of the technical phenomenon and technical progress generates "the technical system", where technology becomes a *milieu*, namely "the new environment in which modern man is required to live" (Ellul 1959: vi).[24] And because it is an environment, it demands nothing else but adaptation.

Therefore, in the time frame of several centuries, technology frees itself from its original ancillary status – which coincides with 'merely' demiurgic-mimetic aspirations – transforming into a completely unprecedented historical event. This happens when man tries to achieve thoroughly one of his innate inclinations: that is, the compensatory and disciplining countermovement regarding his own ek-static tension, the drive of the deficient being that wants to stabilize/immunize the totality of being completely.[25] Such an inclination – which was already expressed by Plato with the definition *"bebaiotes tes ousias"*[26] – expresses the ek-sistence's need to shield its ex-position by concealing the unbearable manifestation of the disclosed open, i.e. the *polemos* which bond world and earth.

The age of technology begins when it becomes *really* (i.e., effectively, *wirklich*) *possible* (i.e., mekeable, *machbar*) to absolutize this compensatory immunizing *pharmakon*, make a whole world of it. As soon as this absolutization occurs, then possibility – which is now reduced only to the possibility of making (something) – becomes cogency and destiny: *"what can be made, must be made"*. Inexorably.[27] The reality is no more *Realität*, nor *Wirklichkeit*, but *Machbarkeit*. "Raw-material-being is *criterium existendi*. Being is being raw material" (Anders 2002b: 33).

Since the open corresponds to the inextricable bond between world and earth, *the age of technology is to be defined as the time when the world swallows up the earth*, i.e. the time of the eclipse of the cosmological difference between world and human world. On the other hand, as we have seen, without earth world cannot exist, and without world, no human world is possible. It follows that the movement triggered by *making technology a world* – "technocosm", technosphere, "technium"[28] – equates to the "de-worldification of the world".[29] With the disappearance of the earth as its *Abgrund*, the world becomes indistinguishable in itself and therefore it plays exactly the same role that the environment has for the animal. The paradoxical outcome of this overall movement is that *technology* (*conceived as a 'universalised* human world') *can achieve a wordly status only in the form of a non-world, that is an environment*: by exhausting man's worldhood, by eroding his ek-statical potentiality. On the other side, this is a completely new type of environment and thus a *neo*-environment.

Now, because man has been characterized on the basis of his 'positional status' – i.e., on the basis of the anthropic perimeter according to: ek-staticity, worldhood, earthhood and historicity – when his natural worldly framework begins to take on environmental features, he experiences an 'animal positionality'. *The main effect of the technological* neoenvironmentality *is the feralization of man. Ipso facto*, this feralization amounts to a liminal situation of anthropology, literally to a post-human threshold, because if (neo)environmentalization were accomplished, man would stop being what he authentically is: a *Weltwesen* (worldly being).

In order to clarify this process, we need to go over the steps we have already described. Since both man's worldhood and animal's environmentality have a pathic focal point – namely, both can be inferred only thanks to those fundamental moods which attune them to their respective findingness – technology has to state its environmental characterisation on a pathic level. As a consequence, our analysis has to go back to its pathic turn. Since animality is characterized by the *Grundstimmung* of captivation (*Benommenheit*), we can attest the feralization of man by identifying traces of such a pathos in his present-day situation. Previously, the peculiarity of the *conditio humana* was attributed to de-severance (*Ent-fernung*): an original distance which prevents man from falling into a complete an immediate fusion with his ecological niche. Given this, an eventual human captivation will have a different genesis from the animal one: it will not correspond to an immediate fact of nature, rather to an effect induced by technological instrumentality, which has achieved the rank of a totality. In other words: it will be a creation of technology, i.e. a product. An artifact.

This unique artifact which is *neoenvironmental captivation* is produced by overexposure, caused by a systematic "calling forth stimulation (*Herausforderung*)" (Heidegger 1953: 14) of which man is the object, and whose "supraliminal" (*überschwellig*) load (Anders 2002a: 262–263 and 1979: 47–48) is for him unbearable because ungraspable, i.e. unexperienceable. The world becomes *overmanned* (Anders 2002b: 26–31) and its calling forth stimulations can only be tolerated by man at the cost of insensivity. That is, in a state of *apatheia*. Pushing to distance from oneself such a type of world, which imposes that integral adaption existing only in the animal *milieu*, becomes impossible. The practice of de-severance is completely inhibited. Unable to carry out his ek-static nature, man finds himself involved in a forced proximity with the world, (con)fused with it and thus enmeshed in it, that is captivated.

The enmeshed stasis of neoenvironmental (con)fusion between man and the world emerges in a deceitful way that already Ernst Jünger called the "total mobilization (*totale Mobilmachung*)" (E. Jünger 1930), i.e. the hysterical dynamism of an endless and purposeless iteration: an epochal framework in which everything moves, but nothing happens.[30] This is a world without history – that is, a world in which technology becomes the "subject of history" – in which man plays the "*co-histori-cal*" role of a mere background actor.[31] A captivated world, and thus a no more world.

As a result, at the peak of his relieving and compensatory trajectory, at the maximum expression of himself as *Kulturwesen* (cultural being), man finds himself in a completely unprecedented situation. Insofar as he is environmentalized (*Umweltwesen* artificially), the inhabitant of tech-nosphere finds himself poor in world, exactly as animal (*Umweltwesen* by nature) is. Deprived of his fundamental capability to de-sever the beings – which is the necessary condition to enter in some relationship with them, to *releasing* them be 'as such' – he impoverishes himself. The decisive premise of the feralization process lies in an *ontological Pauperismus*.[32] In the neoenvironmental cosmos man is reduced to a wholly deficient condition: the *Mangel* of *Mängelwesen* (the deficiency of the deficient being) no longer corresponds to that ontological rich-ness, which is the pure possibility as such, rather it amounts only to shortage, defect and at last, guilt. It becomes ontological debt. Insofar as technology reveals itself as "the organization of a lack (*Mangel*)" (Heidegger 1946: 87), the age of technology proves to be the age of the 'poor in world man': in and for everything a *dürftige Zeit* (time of need).

The logic of *neoenvironmentality* as epochal phenomenon corresponds to the secularized version of a theological dialectics. Being prey of sote-riological anxiety, which is no more psychological but somatic, the feralized man gives birth to a *technodicy*. From the viewpoint of the 'megamachine' (Mumford 1967, Latouche 1995), the human being perceives himself as a permanently defective component because he is never apt to the functions he has been assigned: as much in the field of action (production) as in that of passion (consumption). As some acute interpreters of our time have realized – Debord and Baudrillard in addi-tion to Anders –, the driving force of the present reality is not to be found in production but in consumption, or rather in the production of consumption, i.e. in the production of need. Hence its *phantasmatic, spectacular, simulacral* matrix. Reality becomes the effect of its own projection, the production of its own production and therefore a reproduction. An image. The age of technology is *"The Age of the World Picture (Weltbild)"* (Heidegger 1938), the age of the world reduced to an image. Technocosm is a laboratory of desires, a factory of needs.

Seduced by the phantoms of the "sirenic world" (Anders 2002b: 308–315), the human being commits to a fatal and everlasting attempt to redeem itself from its defectivity, perceived already as guilt. Or, in its secularized version, as a disease. Within such a scenery take shape also the conditions for the adventurous attempts promoted by the variegated constellation of posthumanism. Whose equanimity, its ostentatious ontic horizontality,[33] in fact results in a compulsion to a 'neoenvironmentally correction' of man's intolerable inefficiency (that is, he adapts himself to every demand of the technocosm), so declaring full technological authority and his corresponding minority state. The paradoxical introjection of this imperative according to which we let ourselves be: enhanced, corrected, healed and finally saved from what we ourselves produced, is what Anders defines "Promethean shame", which is the result of the "Promethean gap" that marks "the asynchronicity of the human being with his world of products [...] the inability of our soul to be 'up to date' with our production" (Anders 2002a: 15–16).

The man to come, the post-man, is he who knows how to correspond to all the demands of performances, always new and always increasing, required by the technological neoenvironment.[34] *The ontological Pauperismus, which is the essential cipher of the feralization process, namely of the anthropological metamorphosis (which is potentially post-human) underpinning the phenomenon of neoenvironmentality, is grounded in the defective dogma which produces man's complete having-to-be-made-available of the total mobilization as* homo materia.

Technology, the new *archè kineseos*, represents the essential *pharmakon* for this permanently-in-debt living being, which in order to escape from the condemnation of 'being something' – namely, to give up 'being able to be all that it could be' – forces itself to 'become nothing', i.e. to 'make itself wholly available', recognizing itself as sick and guilty. If the Promethean gap generates the Promethean shame, which increases until it becomes *Promethean guilt*, then in the invocation of technodicy one must root the soteriological anxiety of a *Promethean redemption* from the only mortal sin still present in the Eden of total mobilization: the "*obsolescence*" (*Antiquiertheit*). The aspiration to achieve the condition of a possible post-humanity represents the other side of the coin of obsolescence. Rather than reforming the world to meet human needs and possibilities, it has been chosen to modify man so that he can measure up to a measure-less (overmanned) world. Given such a premise, the human type, which is selected by the technological neoenvironment, will not be a 'simple' *Übermensch*, but a real *Superman*, a post-human subject, namely: 'a-no-longer-only-man'. He is who overcomes the somatic bond expanding it beyond its limits. While breaking the somatic chain used to be the purpose in the past, now the new duty is to extend it (enhance it) indefinitely. The peak, achieved by the totalitarian impulse of neoenvironment, corresponds to the growth of bad conscience inside man, which later becomes Promethean guilt for being 'still only men'. Hence, the following attempt 'to stop being (simply) human'. *The obsolescence is therefore "man's negative attitude towards his being human"*. His *voluptas* for becoming, at last, "sicut machinae" (Anders 2002b: 292).

Given that 'pharmacologic' turns out to be its fundamental vocation, *the essence of technology is thaumaturgic.*[35]

The thaumaturgic outcome of technology, however, marks also the beginning of its ummasking, since it is able to 'free' man only by redeeming itself from its original and fundamental condition: the ancillarity. In order to become a system (a totality), it must transform its servile instrumentality into an end in itself, rise to a *kingdom of means*. "Having become a *universum* of means and media, technology is in fact the environment of man" (Ellul 1980: 38).[36] This occurs, as we have seen, if technology becomes world, namely if world becomes environment. And the world environmentalizes itself only on condition that man ceases to be aware himself *as such*, i.e. if he attunes himself to the mood of captivation. Neoenvironmental *Benommenheit* – an *insensitivity to the earth*, which is equivalent to a condition of integral circumspection (*Umsicht*) – becomes really possible when it becomes really impossible to interrupt the *Alltäglichkeit* circuit, that is when technology becomes able to totally inhibit the *thauma* (the earthly *Stimmung* brought about by the disclosure of the open), making of it, from the *pathos* that it is, an *ergon*, i.e. a product, an artifact.

'Technically creating *thauma*', namely: producing it, making it happen, implementing it, is quite literally 'thauma-thurgy' (*thauma* + *ergon*). So such a process represents the fundamental thaumaturgic aim of technology, its paradoxical soteriological aspiration.[37]

Nevertheless thaumaturge is and remains a magician by definition.[38] Just insofar as thaumaturgy corresponds to: *induction, production, challenge* of the wonder, it is an artifice, a *mechanè*. A trick. The basic trick that this *pharmakon* needs in order to bestow its healing virtues lies in our distorted belief in considering as infinite possibilities those things that are, on the contrary, only infinite modes of adaptation made preventively available (fore-cast) by the technosphere. To be successful, this trick makes use of our illusion to consider ourselves as free and all-powerful, while at the same time we give ourselves up to the impotence of formlessness, the limitation of instrumental adaptation giving up the use of our ek-static potentiality. As said: we make ourselves nothing, in order not to be 'only' something.

This means that thaumaturgy can try to produce *thauma*, and so annihilate it *as such*, only by falsifying it. By making it what it cannot be, because as fundamental pathos it cannot be either called forth or produced. *Thauma* equates to the reaction to a surplus, which is in itself ungraspable and thus irreducible to any human measure. Therefore any possible production and calling forth stimulation (*Herausforderung*) has to presuppose it. The only sign of its presence is the wondering horror that it causes in that particular being that is able to be aware of it by being aware of itself. This particular being can disclose itself to the disclosure (open) by recognizing (i.e., feeling) that he is situated, exposed in such a disclosure. Because man is this same ex-position, he is essentially a correspondence, a response to the call of that disclosure (open). Just by being there, he finds himself beyond the reach of what neoenvironmental captivation would bring back to itself by artifacting it. There is no way to go back to such an origin, to call forth that call to which we are inevitable the response. We can only try to remove it with a trick, i.e. inhibiting our capability to be aware of it. As a consequence, it is not given a real eclipse of cosmological difference, because it is not given world which swallows the earth: world can only conceal it with a conjurer's trick.

So thaumaturgy – the current *telos* of *techne* – turns out to be an illusion and a trick. It equates to man's highest (but completely unrealistic) irresponsibility not to wish to assume his own response, i.e. the correspondence that he himself is. On the other hand, this irresponsibility itself represents a response to that call from which man would like to escape by silencing it. Even beyond the mask of neoenvironmental feralization, hides a *Weltwesen*.

Postscript. The Humanity of the Posthuman

" . . . the philosophical abstraction, regardless of normal and habitual circumspection [...] With this examining without any particular intention, simply for love of understanding, philosophying begins as *theorein* without an aim (*zweckloses* theorein)" (Löwith 1960: 315). These words, which summarize the basic inspiration of Löwith's cosmocentric anthropology (Cera 2010 and 2013: 81–146), relate man's peculiarity and consequent anthropological difference to the distinction between two fundamental *pathic functions*: contemplation (*Betrachtung*) and circumspection (*Umsicht*).

Man is worldly being (*Weltwesen*), but he is worldly in that he is (potentially) *capable* of that fundamental pathos that allows him to experience the cosmological difference between world and human world. *Theorein* (contemplation) is such a pathic function. But, as we said, contemplation corresponds to the disciplining of a more original pathos: *thauma/thaumazein* (the 'wondering horror'). It follows that *man is in effect worldly in that he is potentially contemplative.* *Weltwesen* is essentially *Betrachtungswesen*: the being of contemplation and wondering.

The animal, on its side, is environmental being (*Umweltwesen*), but it is environmental in that it is *characterized* (actually) by that fundamental pathos which does not allow it to experience any cosmological difference. Circumspection, namely instrumental and self-absorbed behavior, is such a pathic function. But, as we said, circumspection is the effect of a more deeply rooted captivation/enmeshment, which causes animal's (con)fusion with its own ecological niche. *The animal is in effect environmental in that it is actually* (cogently) *circumspect, i.e. captivated*. The *Umweltwesen* is apparently an *Umsichtswesen* (a being of circumspection), but it is essentially a *Benommenheitswesen* (a being of captivation).

The potential aspect of man's worldly pathos is such that it can be referred at least partly to his free responsibility. 'Being human' means also 'becoming human' and staying as such. As Helmuth Plessner stated, *hominitas* is not yet *humanitas* (Plessner 1956). The fulfillment of our *Bestimmung* (determination and destination) carries with it a duty and a task, so that an anthropology with philosophical ambitions involves naturally an intrinsic ethical component. The fact that being human is a task to be carried out implies the possibility of its failure, too. In such a circumstance, there would be the paradoxical result of having a hypothetical *conditio post-humana* entirely identical to the animal condition, i.e. man would become unrecognizable to his own eyes. This is exactly what this essay wishes to say. *According to the neoenvironmental hypothesis* – in terms of which technology, raised to the rank of phenomenon and system, produces a posthuman threshold by eroding the anthropic perimeter – *posthuman pathos emerges as an artificial*

Benommenheit *triggered by the systematic inhibition of the* dynamis theoretica, *i.e. the authentic worldly pathos.* As a consequence, the post-man (that is, the man who is completely adapted to the technological neoenvironment) will correspond to the perfectly circumspect man, or rather the thoroughly rationalised man ('the integral rational agent'), who can no longer get out from his instrumental vital circle because he is enmeshed, captivated in it.

When technology manages to dictate this pseudo-captivation to man, it becomes what the environment is for the animal: it demands a complete and immediate adaption. As a consequence, while technology becomes environment, on the other side man accomplishes his feraliza-tion. The inhibition of his *dynamis theoretica* ferinizes him, but according to a peculiar way. Differently from the animal – whose environmentalization is the outcome of integral circumspection produced by its fundamental captivation – man becomes a totally environmental being in that he is completely captivated, but completely captivated in that he is wholly circumspect. In other words, he is *Umweltwesen* in that he is *Umsichtswesen*.

In the age of fulfilled secularization, the duty of determining ourselves is entirely our responsibility. Paradoxically, the real *hybris* of the posthuman technolatry is such not because it is too much, rather it is too little, namely, it is an insatiable will to delegate. So the real definition of the posthuman age is to be found not in "Wille zur Macht" (Will to power), but in unmentionably *Wille zum Gemacht* (Will to be made) or, as previously said, in *"man's negative attitude towards his being human"*.

Despite its ostentatious claims to activism, the spirit of the posthuman ideology seems to promote a *de facto* abdication of the basic directives that our condition has always imposed on us. It encourages a depreciated *Gelassenheit*, a kind of *regressus ad hominitatem*, a downgrading from *humanitas* to *hominitas* with its blind commitment to technology, letting us be manipulated by it *ad libitum*. All this is accompanied by the naïve soteriological hope that what technology 'wants' will be necessarily our own good.

The fact that humanity is always the outcome of a never-ending historical process and not an atemporal datum does not make it unworthy of being defended and safeguarded. Just waiting to see what it will make of us, would be a legitimate conduct within a fideistic and creationist context, but not certainly at the peak of the *secular age*. More so because technology, in that it is instrumentality, is by definition atelic and ateleonomic, i.e. incapable of establishing any authentic purpose.

The actual post-human/neoenvironmental arrogance lies in its pretension that it can release us from the load that we ourselves are. Instead, what our age urgently requires is that we really take on the responsibility to ourselves, by addressing now our future condition, since what we will be depends mostly on what we will choose to be. Keeping in mind, in making this choice, that nowadays as always the authentic dignity of our *Bestimmung* depends not only on always reaching the goal of 'what we have not been yet', but in our capability to recognize and safeguard 'what we can worthily continue being'.

Notes

1 (moonwatch1@libero.it Department of Human Sciences (DISU) – University of Basilicata – Potenza, Italy).

2 For the content as much as for the complete bibliography, see first and foremost Cera (2013, especially: 147–192), where the 'neoenvironmentality hypothesis' is first formulate in its entirety, and then Cera (2007 and 2012).

3 Assuming, with respect to the question of animality and anthropological difference, a position which relates to von Uexküll's reflections re-read in the Heideggerian sense, we also take into account Derrida's criticisms, in his attempt (unfortunately unfinished) to rethink animality and the animal on the basis of its being renamed "*animot*" (Derrida 2008). Giorgio Agamben starts from a comparison between the animal condition (environmental) and the human (worldly), this too inspired by Heidegger's reflections, in order to develop a hypothesis which presents objective elements of proximity with that of *neoenvironmentality* (Agamben 2004).

4 "I refuse to present my thinking in the form of a theory or in a systematic fashion. I am making a dialectical ensemble that is open and not closed and I am making sure not to present solutions of the ensemble [...] If I did do these things, I too would be contributing to the technological totalization." (Ellul 1980: 204n).

5 Many other names could be added. For example: the first exponents of the Frankfurt School, then Oswald Spengler, Ernst Cassirer and, more recently, Andrew Feenberg, Gilbert Hottois, Carl Mitcham, Emanuele Severino and Bernard Stiegler. For a brief historical *excursus* of the philosophy of technology, see Hottois (2003: 13–23) and Cera (2007: 44–67).

6 As is well known, the idea of an *anthropotechnics* is discussed by Peter Sloterdijk (Sloterdijk 2013). In the context of posthumanism, Roberto Marchesini proposes the "*antropo-poiesi*" formula, as the outcome of the process of "anthropodecentrism" (Marchesini 2002 and 2009: 80–86).

7 "L'inizio, per quell'esserci che sa di averlo, è nel suo saperlo" (Mazzarella 2004: 13).

8 For engineering and neo-engineering approaches to *technology*, see Cera (2007: 52–56, 63–67).

9 In the famous (Löwith 1957), Karl Löwith finds the congenital defect of the philosophy of history in its undue transformation from universal history (*Weltgeschichte*) to the advent of salvation (*Heilsgeschehen*). Some exam-

ples of such a decline of the diagnostic capacity because of excessive prog-
nostic aspirations are to be found in some passages in the later works of
Ellul (1980 and 1990).

10 The concept of 'worldhood' put forward here presents some analogies with
the "worldhood" (*Weltlichkeit*) of *Being and Time* (Heidegger 2001: 91–
123). As for Uexküll's *Umweltlehre*, this is assumed on the basis of a
rereading by Gehlen (1988) and especially Heidegger (1995).

11 The most significant antecedents of this positional approach to philosophical anthropology are those of Scheler (who translates the question of man
into that of determination of his place 'in the cosmos'), followed by Plessner
who thinks of man in terms of (eccentric) 'positionality' (Scheler 2009,
Plessner 1981).

12 "The 'milieu' (*Umgebung*) is the set of those elements in a vital space,
connected to each other by the laws of nature, the space in which we observe
the organism [...] 'environment' (*Umwelt*) is the set of those conditions
contained in the whole complex of a *milieu* which allow a certain organism
to survive thanks to its specific organization [...] the concept of environment so defined is difficult to apply to man [...] we cannot point to a specific
environment or a *milieu* to which he could be assigned in the sense of the
preceding definition." (Gehlen 1942: 79–80).

13 Uexküll writes with reference to the animal: "everything a subject perceives
belongs to its *perception world* (Merkwelt), and everything it produces, to
its *effect world* (Wirkwelt). These two worlds, of perception and production
of effects, form one closed unit, the *environment* (Umwelt)." (Uexküll 2010:
42). By Uexküll we have to mention at least (Uexküll 1921), the work with
which Heidegger dialogues directly in (Heidegger 1995).

14 A little earlier, he reiterates the difference of conditions – which do not hierarchical – between man and animal: "As far as the animal is concerned we
cannot say that beings are closed off from it. Beings could only be closed
off if there were some possibility of disclosure at all [...] the captivation
(*Benommenheit*) of the animal places the animal essentially outside of the
possibility that beings could be either disclosed to it or closed off from it."
(Heidegger 1995: 248).

15 In his discussion of the topic of animality, (Buchanan 2008) proposes an
onto-ethological approach.

16 In (Anders 1937) this intrinsic distance of man from the world
(*Weltfremdheit*) is described in terms of freedom. This is unconsciously in
agreement with Gehlen's position, in which estrangement (*Entfremdung*)
represents the genetic nucleus of freedom (Gehlen 1952).

17 For the concept of "relief", see (Gehlen 1988: 54–64). For that of "de-severance", reference has been made to § 23 of *Being and Time*, where Heidegger
defines *de-severance* (*Ent-fernung*), as well as *directionality* (*Ausrichtung*),
the building blocks of spatiality of Dasein: "'*De-severing*' amounts to
making the *farness* vanish – that is, making the *remoteness* of something
disappear, bringing it close. Dasein is essentially *de-severant*." (Heidegger
2001: 139, my italics).

18 For the concept of *Weltfremdheit* see Anders (1937), which in the original

german version (now lost) was entitled *Die Weltfremdheit des Menschen*. For that of *Weltoffenheit* see Scheler (2009).

19 On the subject of the cosmological difference between world and human world, see Löwith (1960) and Cera (2013: 81–146).

20 This description presents a clear analogy with the mystifying idea of nature expressed by Uexküll: "Forever unknowable behind all of the worlds it produces, the subject – Nature – conceals itself." (Uexküll 2010: 135).

21 It is in fact its passive, reactive character which makes of the pathic sphere – in contrast to the *praxis* and the *ergon* – a dimension, which is not entirely within-the-world and therefore a potential ek-static bridge which leads from the world to the earth. On this topic see Cera (2013: 167–192).

22 Ex-position corresponds to the 'fundamental situation' of the human being when wholly revealed, i.e. his being within the open of *polemos* between world and earth. The *thauma* represents the tell-tale echo of such an ex-position. Nevertheless pure ex-position is in itself dazzling and therefore unbearable. In order to make it bearable the filter of a minimum distance is needed. This filter marks already the imposing of the discipline of *logos*: that which makes *thauma* (the wondering horror) *thaumazein* (wonder, marvel) and then *theorein* (detached contemplation). In this sense, the very famous philosophical genesis narrated by Aristotle (*Metaphysics* I, 2, 982b), and before him by Plato (*Thaetetus* 155d), proves to be incomplete, because the birth of philosophy does come from the working of wonder (*thaumazein*), but the latter is essentially transfiguration and concealment of horror (*thauma*).

23 In a famous passage of his *Tractatus* (6.44), Wittgenstein expressed *the mystical* (das Mystische) exactly in these terms: "Nicht *wie* die Welt is, ist das Mystische, sondern *dass* sie ist (not *how* the world is, is the mystical, but *that* it is)." (Wittgenstein 1922: 89).

24 On technique as man's *milieu*, see also chapter two of Ellul (1980: 34–51), entitled: *Technology as an Environment*.

25 On discipline as a necessary compensation for *Mängelwesen*, see Gehlen (1988: 351–364). More in general, on the concept of "compensation" in philosophical anthropology, see Marquard (1983).

26 Plato, *Cratylus* 386a 3–4.

27 "*Not only is it a rule that what can be made* (das Gekonnte) *must be made* (das Gesollte), *but also that what must be made is inevitable* (das Unvermeidliche)" (Anders 2002b: 17). This is Anders's re-reading of the so-called 'law of Gabor', formulated by the Hungarian physicist Dennis Gabor in (Gabor 1972).

28 Sharing Ellul's hypothesis for a systemic interpretation of technology, Gilbert Hottois speaks of "technocosme" or "règne technique" (Hottois 1984). Taking recourse to the neologism "technium", Kevin Kelly recognizes the systemic characterization of contemporary technology, but in a totally apologetic way. His work is a catechetical handbook, put together to facilitate adaptation (conversion) to the neoenvironment (Kelly 2010).

29 Using the formula "Entweltlichung der Welt" Löwith describes the overall parabola of modernity (*Neuzeit*), which in his reconstruction wholly coincides with Christian metaphysics (Löwith 1967: 10).

30 Of course, this is a purposelessness that has nothing to do with the atelic gratuity of the *theorein*. The being without purpose in this case corresponds to the extreme form of the extreme interest: to the sum of whole circumspection.

31 In the context of a general "a-historicity" (*Ungeschichtlichkeit*), decreed by the rise of technology as "subject of history" (*Subjekt der Geschichte*), Günther Anders speaks of a man's regression to a "co-historical" (*mitgeschichtlich*) condition (Anders 2002b: 9, 271–278).

32 "Every rationalization is the consequence of scarcity. The expansion and constant perfection of the technical apparatus are not merely the result of the technician's urge for power; they are just as much the result of want. This is why the human situation characteristic of our machine world is poverty (*Pauperismus*). And this poverty cannot be overcome by any technological efforts." (F. G. Jünger 1956: 13).

33 Roberto Marchesini (2009: 16–18) speaks of *"horizontality of* bios". Nevertheless such a horizontality seems to be achieved at the cost of a preliminary gesture of indifference: the reduction of living beings to the rank of a material available to the 'needs' of technology.

34 Byung-Chul Han describes the 21th century as a "perfomance society" (*Leistungsgesellschaft*), whose components are "subjects of performance" (*Leistungssubjekte*). See (Han 2015: 8).

35 By affirming this, we intend to maintain that the everyday characterization of pauperism as a vehicle of neoenvironmental enmeshment is the *pathologization*. Technological thaumaturgy trains pathos, making it pathology (disease) and so promoting its self-censorship. Once we have recognized ourselves as being 'pathic', we perceive ourselves as being 'sick', defective. And finally guilty. That is: we are ready to become devotees of technological soteriology. On this topic, see Cera (2012: 38–45).

36 In order to explain the expression 'universum of means' the following passage by Umberto Galimberti can be useful: "if the technological means is the necessary condition to achieve any aim which cannot be achieved without technological means, the achievement of the means becomes the real aim which subordinates everything to itself" (Galimberti 2004: 37).

37 On the holy and religious dimension of technology see Noble (1997) and Davis (1998).

38 Plato attributes the sophist, a technician *par excellence,* to the "*genos ton thaumatopoion*", the genus of conjurors (*Sophist* 235b 5). In Ancient Greece, the *thaumatourgoi* were the constructors of *thaumata*: those special machines which entertained audiences by 'making wonder'. On this topic, see Cambiano (2006).

Bibliography

Accarino, B. 1991: Tra libertà e decisione: alle origini dell'antropologia filosofica. In B. Accarino (ed.), *Ratio Imaginis. Uomo e mondo nell'antropologia filosofica*. Firenze: Ponte alle Grazie, 7–63.

Agamben, G. 2004: *The Open: Man and Animal*, trans. K. Attell. Stanford: Stanford University Press.

Anders, G. 1935: Une interprétation de l'a posteriori. *Recherches philosophiques*, IV (1934/1935), 65–80.

Anders, G. 1937: Pathologie de la libérte. *Recherches philosophiques*, VI (1936/1937), 22–54.

Anders, G. 1979: Wenn ich verzweifelt bin, was geht's mich an? Gespräch mit Günther Anders. In M. Greffrath (ed.), *Die Zerstörung einer Zukunft. Gespräche mit emigrierten Sozialwissenschaftlern*. Hamburg: Rowohlt, 19–57.

Anders, G. 2002a: *Die Antiquiertheit des Menschen 1. Über die Seele im Zeitalter der zweiten industriellen Revolution*. München: Beck.

Anders, G. 2002b: *Die Antiquiertheit des Menschen 2. Über die Zerstörung des Lebens im Zeitalter der dritten industriellen Revolution*. München: Beck.

Buchanan, B. 2008: *Onto-ethologies. The Animal Environments of Uexküll, Heidegger, Merleau-Ponty and Deleuze*. Albany: SUNY Press.

Cambiano, G. 2006: Automaton. In *Figure, macchine, sogni. Saggi sulla scienza antica*. Roma: Edizioni di Storia e Letteratura, 175–196.

Cera, A. 2007: Sulla questione di una filosofia della tecnica. In N. Russo (ed.), *L'uomo e le macchine. Per un'antropologia della tecnica*. Napoli: Guida, 41–115.

Cera, A. 2010: *Io con tu. Karl Löwith e la possibilità di una Mitanthropologie*. Napoli: Guida.

Cera, A. 2012: Il metron della techne. Apologia della diserzione. *Etica & Politica* XIV (1), 27–45.

Cera, A. 2013: *Tra differenza cosmologica e neoambientalità. Sulla possibilità di un'antropologia filosofica oggi*. Napoli: Giannini.

Davis, E. 1998: *Techgnosis. Myth, Magic, and Mysticism in the Age of Information*. New York: Harmony Books.

Derrida, J. 2008: *The Animal That Therefore I Am*, trans. M.-L. Mallet. New York: Fordham University Press.

Ellul, J. 1959, Presentazione dell'Autore all'edizione italiana. In *La tecnica, rischio del secolo*, trad. it. C. Pesce, Milano: Giuffrè.

Ellul, J. 1964: *The Technological Society*, trans. J. Wilkinson. New York: Vintage Books.

Ellul, J. 1980: *The Technological System*, trans. J. Neugroschel. New York: Continuum.

Ellul, J. 1990: *The Technological Bluff*, trans. G. W. Bromiley. Grand Rapids (Michigan): Eerdmans.

Ellul, J. 1984: Tecnica. in *Enciclopedia del Novecento Treccani*. http://goo.gl/KjjOE0

Gabor, D. 1972: *The Mature Society*. New York: Praeger.

Galimberti, U. 2004: *Psiche e techne. L'uomo nell'età della tecnica*. Milano: Feltrinelli.

Gehlen, A. 1942: Zur Systematik der Anthropologie. In *Philosophische Anthropologie und Handlungslehre, Gesamtausgabe Band 4*, hrsg. von K.-S. Rehberg. Frankfurt am Main: Klostermann, 63–112.

Gehlen, A. 1952: Über die Geburt der Freiheit aus der Entfremdung. In *Philosophische Anthropologie und Handlungslehre*, 366–379.

Gehlen, A. 1988: *Man. His Nature and Place in the World*, trans. C. McMillan and K. Pillemer. New York: Columbia University Press.

Han, B.-Ch. 2015: *The Burnout Society*, trans. E. Butler. Stanford: Stanford University Press.

Heidegger, M. 1929: On the Essence of Ground. In *Pathmarks*, trans. W. McNeill. Cambridge/New York: Cambridge University Press 1998, 97–135.

Heidegger, M. 1936: The Origin of the Work of Art. In *Off the Beaten Track*, trans. J. Young and K. Haynes. Cambridge: Cambridge University Press 2002, 1–56.

Heidegger, M. 1938: The Age of the World Picture. In *Off the Beaten Track*, 57–85.

Heidegger, M. 1946: Overcoming Metaphysics. In R. Wolin (ed.), *The Heidegger Controversy: A Critical Reader*. Cambridge/London: The MIT Press 1998, 67–90.

Heidegger, M. 1953: The Question Concerning Technology. In *The Question Concerning Technology and Other Essays*, trans. W. Lovitt. New York & London: Garland 1977, 3–35.

Heidegger, M. 1995: *The Fundamental Concepts of Metaphysics. World, Finitude, Solitude*, trans. W. McNeill and N. Walker. Bloomington and Indianapolis: Indiana University Press.

Heidegger, M. 2001: *Being and Time*, trans. J. Macquarrie and E. Robinson. Oxford: Blackwell.

Hottois, G. 1984: *Le signe et la technique. La philosophie a l'épreuve de la technique*. Paris: Aubier.

Hottois, G. 2003: Les philosophes et la technique. Les philosophes de la technique. In G. Hottois and P. Chabot (eds), *Les philosophes et la technique*. Paris: Vrin, 13–23.

Jünger, E. 1930: Total Mobilization. In R. Wolin (ed.), *The Heidegger Controversy: A Critical Reader*, 118–139.

Jünger, F. G. 1956: *The Failure of Technology. Perfection Without Purpose*, trans. F. D. Wilhelmsen. Chicago: Regnery.

Latouche, S. 1995: *La mégamachine. Raison techno-scientifique, raison économique et mythe du progrès. Essais à la mémoire de Jacques Ellul*. Paris: La Découverte.

Löwith, K. 1957: *Meaning in History. The Theological Implications of the Philosophy of History*. Chicago/London: Chicago University Press.

Löwith, K. 1960: Welt und Menschenwelt. In *Sämtliche Schriften Band 1*, hrsg. von K. Stichweh. Stuttgart: Metzler, 295–328.

Löwith, K. 1967: Gott, Mensch und Welt in der Metaphysik von Descartes bis zu Nietzsche. In *Sämtliche Schriften Band 9*, hrsg. von H. Ritter. Stuttgart: Metzler 1–194.

Marchesini, R. 2002: *Post-human. Verso nuovi modelli di esistenza*. Torino: Bollati Boringhieri.

Marchesini, R. 2009: *Il tramonto dell'uomo. La prospettiva post-umanista*. Bari: Dedalo.

Marquard, O. 1983: Homo compensator. Zur anthropologischen Karriere eines metaphysischen Begriffs. In *Philosophie des Stattdessen*. Stuttgart: Reclam 2000, 11–29.

Mazzarella, E. 2004: *Vie d'uscita. L'identità umana come programma stazio-nario metafisico*. Genova: il melangolo.

Mumford, L. 1967: *The Myth of The Machine 1. Technics and Human Development*. New York: Harcourt, Brace & World.

Noble, D. F. 1997: *The Religion of Technology. The Divinity of Man and the Spirit of Invention*. New York: Knopf.

Plessner, H. 1956: Über einige Motive der Philosophischen Anthropologie. In *Gesammelte Schriften VIII*, hrsg. von G. Dux u.a. Frankfurt am Main: Suhrkamp 1983, 117–135.

Plessner, H. 1981: Die Stufen des Organischen und der Mensch. Einleitung in die philosophische Anthropologie. In *Gesammelte Schriften IV*, hrsg. von G. Dux u.a. Frankfurt am Main: Suhrkamp 1981.

Scheler, M. 2009: *The Human Place in the Cosmos*, trans. M. Frings. Evanston (Illinois): Northwestern University Press.

Sloterdijk, P. 2013: *You Must Change Your Life. On Anthropotechnics*, trans. W. Hoban. Cambridge: Polity.

Uexküll von, J. 2010: A Foray into the World of Animals and Humans. In *A Foray into the World of Animals and Humans. With a Theory of Meaning*, trans. J. D. O'Neil. Minneapolis/London: University of Minnesota Press, 41–135.

Uexküll von, J. 1921: *Umwelt und Innenwelt der Tiere*, (zweite vermehrte und verbesserte Auflage). Berlin/Heidelberg: Springer.

Volpi, F. 2004: *Il nichilismo*. Roma-Bari: Laterza.

Wittgenstein, L. 1922: *Tractatus Logico-Philosophicus*, trans. C. K. Ogden. London/New York: Trubner & Co./Harcourt, Brace & Co.

12

Emotive Bond With Machines (or Through Machines)

Paolo Gallina

Why do we have emotions? Why, when my daughter wants to play at two o'clock at night, is her smile enough not to make me want to throw her out of the window? Why does a child beggar almost always manage to make me fork out a euro? And how is it that, with a caress and a few sweet words, my wife gets me to holiday in the mountains when I am in no way fond of the mountains?

Our emotions, or rather the emotions involved in social relationships, exist in order to make people do things they would otherwise not do.

The emotions were created by nature to enable man to live in small communities such as the family or larger social units like a village, a town or a state. They are not glue. They exist to encourage altruistic behaviour. If a person were assimilated into a crowd free to move on the plain, emotions would be the forces that push the crows in a precise direction. Other forces are set against these, forces of an egocentric nature such as the survival instinct, the necessity to satisfy primary and secondary needs, the need to escape pain, the drive to search for personal pleasure, and so on.

It is from the dynamics, and above all the equilibrium of our emotions set off against our individualistic instincts, that society as we know it takes its form. In making every daily choice, the mind puts on the scales the weights of *I* and *others* and works out a result which is translated into a concrete action. This is why the emotions, apart from being the salt of life, are from the biological point of view decisional tools.

The emotions possess two basic characteristics that make them effective: they are *irrational* and *immediate*.

This statement contains a paradox that can be summarized in the question: How can irrationality make a mental process effective? It is usually believed that a choice made on the basis of irrational reasoning is almost always wrong, or at least, not the best one. However, this is not statistically true, especially if the time variable is taken into consideration. In order to see how true this is, we can think back to my first question, the one about my daughter wanting to play at two o'clock at night, and ask ourselves what a character like Mr. Spock, the ultimate in the rational without emotion, would have done in my place. The Vulcan would have thought that his body was tired and that he should have been in bed a long time ago, otherwise the day after he would not have been able to pilot the Enterprise properly. However, he would also have taken into consideration the fact that one day the child would be a woman, would herself have a child, and so increased the likelihood of the human being's survival. Furthermore, he would have considered the fact that the child was not asleep because she had slept during the day. He would then have assessed the psychological harm to the child if he had made her cry because he did not play with her, harm caused by her sense of being abandoned in the middle of the night, and increased by her fear of darkness. Furthermore . . . After a hundred or so 'furthermores', and so after half an hour of reasoning, Mr. Spock would have decided to play with the child.

Coincidentally, this is the same decision that I myself take every time I find myself in this situation. The point is, however, that I cannot afford to spend half an hour in quantitative analysis, assessing the pros and cons, every time I am required to make a choice involving another human being. Life is too short for it. And so we have an explanation for the other main characteristic of the emotions: their immediacy.

To dismiss the leading role of the emotions because of their irrational structure is a wrong. The emotions have been refined and modified throughout evolution so that all of us can make use of them to reach common objectives. In other words, the irrational emotions of every individual are the result of rationality stripped of natural emotion.

The emotions, therefore, are similar to a consultant. This consultant is always present in our minds, they point to the direction we should take without going into the reasons and evaluations supporting their suggestion. The consultant encourages us to rock a crying baby (thanks to affection), it stops us from reprimanding a colleague too severely when he has made a mistake (thanks to empathy), it forces us to listen more carefully to a beautiful girl simply because she is beautiful (thanks to attraction), etc. But above all, this consultant makes its suggestions in an extraordinarily short time. The emotions have one more basic characteristic which we should remember: *they are never disabled*. Not even by a rational thought which attempts to oppose them.

I dislike the memory of my terrifying exam in Machines and Mechanical Engineering. The professor sat on his chair with a bulldog expression and barked in silence. I stood at the blackboard with a stub of chalk in my sweating, trembling fingers. My heart was beating madly. And my throat felt like sandpaper. I had done everything within my power to stay calm and not allow myself to be intimidated by the professor's glaring eyes. I had tried imagining him sitting in his pants on the toilet, tried telling myself that an exam is nothing compared to a road accident, I had played the card of rationality: however badly it went, what harm could the professor do me? Break my arm? No, of course not, he could only tell me to come back and try again. And yet, for all the mental commitment spent in trying to analyses the situation rationally, that overwhelming sensation of inhibition remained throughout the exam. All of us have many such experiences, experiences in which we would like to mitigate or modify in some way the unconscious working of the emotions. Unfortunately, our reason is unable always to overcome the emotions. As we shall see, this property is fundamental when we move from an analysis of the emotions felt for a human being to those felt with regard to a machine.

1. Taking it Out on Your Bicycle

Have you ever taken it out on your punctured bicycle by kicking it? Or shaken your mobile phone because it wouldn't work? Or hurled insults at the recorded voice at a motorway toll gate after hours waiting in the queue? Of course you have. Objects, and especially machines, sometimes seem to do all they can to make life difficult. They can seem mean, even wicked. But above all, for some fractions of a second, they seem to have a will of their own, a kind of soul able to knowingly alter the events of life. Obviously, once we have let off steam, reason takes us back to reality and reminds us that an inanimate object is not sentient and has no will of its own.

The fact remains that there are some situations in which machines manage to trigger emotions resembling those inspired by interaction with other living beings.

If we then move from the simple sphere of inanimate objects to that of digital systems, from robotics to artificial intelligence, the phenomenon of the generation of feelings that may be defined *artificial emotions* reaches dimensions and an intensity that are anything but negligible. So much so that industry has for some time realized their persuasive effects, using them scientifically in order to increase profits.

Why – and the question relates the emotional properties of machines to the area of interest of this essay – are some machines able to cheat our minds, "extorting" emotions that we have no real reason to feel?

The explanation is to be sought in the very nature of man, a nature that began to be forged in prehistory, a long way away from technological influences. As we saw above, emotions are irrational, immediate and cannot be deactivated. We also saw that immediacy has a distinct advantage in terms of behavioural strategies in that it enables us to take a decision in the shortest possible time and certainly a shorter interval of time than that which is necessary to follow a rational argument knowingly to its end.

But at double the price: on the one hand the emotions produce impulsive actions which at times are not appropriate to their context; on the other, in order to be reactive, the expression of emotion is based on little information. The face of a child is enough to move us, and not the child as a whole. A warm voice on the telephone is enough to reassure us, and not the actual person on the line. A frown and tight lips on a severe face are more than enough to induce uneasiness without the owner of the eyes and lips doing or saying anything remotely accusing. And if, at night, the wind shakes a curtain making it look as if it might be a burglar, before we starting looking for logical explanations, we are invaded by terror.

Inevitably, the thing which triggers emotion – the emotion that any human being feels in response to another human being – is an incomplete and approximate representation of the object of that emotion. In other words, it is the image, movement, voice and other incomplete details of a person that makes us feel emotion and not the person in himself.

A machine cannot and will never be identical to a human being. However, it can imitate certain of the human's characteristics: the face, movements, voice and overall shape. And it is by virtue of these partial, incomplete representations that, under certain conditions, a machine can become the active generator of artificial emotions.

2. Computers Which Generate Emotion

To look more closely at the matter, moving from abstraction to concrete observation, we should look at digital technology. Is the computer simply a machine which helps us carry out certain functions, or one which has properties that transcend its particular structure? It is tempting to reply that it is only a tool, the outcome of the assembling of electromechanical parts lacking any spark of life. This is what reason tells us. But, as we have seen, reason and emotion do not always arrive at the same conclusion. In the nineties, the sociologist Clifford Nass and his collaborators attempted to look into the dynamics of reason and emotion using a scientific, quantitative approach. They had an idea for, and carried out, a series of experiments in which a statistically significant number of subjects were asked to interact with a number of computers.

In one of these experiments, perhaps the most famous, computers with "diversified communicative styles and characteristics" were used. 41 subjects were divided into three groups and asked to interact with three computers programmed to respond to questions in a precise and predetermined way. Each of the subjects had to cooperate with the computer in carrying out a task by means of a kind of interaction that involved using the screen and the keyboard. The computers asked question to which the subjects – if they felt they should – had to reply. The first group did not receive any particular feedback from the computer. The subjects of the second group, however, received gratifying feedback in the form of a compliment after every question. In this case the subject had been told beforehand that the computer would give praise independently of the quality of the reply. The subjects of the third group received the same identical feedback as that of the second group, but were not told beforehand about the 'praising' behaviour of the machine. The results were unequivocal: the subjects of the second and third groups, compared to those of the first, showed greater appreciation of the experiment, a greater desire to continue the work and, above all, they judged the quality of their performance favourably (Fogg and Nass 1997). The conclusions of the experiment shows that "artificial praise" in man-to-computer interaction produce effects resembling those in man-to-man interactions.

Another pioneer of research on the dynamics of interaction with digital technologies, B.J. Fogg, in a paper explaining how machines can influence their users, describes computers that interact with man as *social actors*, that is systems able to "recite", according to various modalities and nuances, a role which competes with man and his social behavior (Fogg 2002). According to Fogg, the "skeleton keys" that the computer uses to create an irrational emotional contact are physicality, psychology, language, social dynamics roles. Physicality is implemented by the use of avatars or characters anthropomorphized with agents, able to transmit the sensation that "inside" the computer there is a human presence. A well-known example is Clippy, the likeable sexless assistant of Office, now no longer used, in the shape of a paper clip with lively eyes. Clippy had no specific task to carry out other than hop about and wink at the right moment, actions which were intended to create a bond of complicity with the user. All to make more tolerable the interface between graphics and commands which were not yet optimized and therefore complex.

Psychological aspects are the most important ingredients to be dominated in opening an emotive channel of communication between man and computer. In my work as a university lecturer, when I am obliged to fail a student at exams, I avoid using words such as "You have not studied well enough. Come back next time." I am inclined to communicate the bad news with a certain amount of tact: "I'm sorry, you are not well prepared enough for this exam. You will have to repeat it." In our families, at work, even when we go out to buy bread, the amount of information we communicate to others is only a part of the set of information transmitted. Our style of introducing ourselves to a stranger, our farewells, our uses of the conditionals, are forms of courtesy which are needed to open an emotive channel. In financial transactions this channel is just as important as the sales price. And given that many information structures have been devised in order to implement financial transactions, it seems evident that these tend to implement and reproduce psychological schemata by borrowing them from man's social processes.

In this respect, it is possible to equip computers with a personality which is sufficiently well-defined and discernable. The *principle of similarity* suggests that it is easier to accept the advice and opinions of those whose characters resemble our own. The unassertive truest the unassertive and distrust troublemakers. Decisions are made with respect to points of view expressed strongly. The irresolute are ready to accept truths expressed with a certain degree of uncertainty. The same rules apply to computers. Domineering subjects prefer to work (and perform better) with software whose claims and schemes are domineering. The opposite is true of submissive subjects with a noticeable sense of insecurity (Gouldner 1960).

The principle of similarity also appertains to belonging to a group or a society. It is a phenomenon which, quite apart from the case of computers, we experience every day. Members of the same political alliance show greater willingness to exchange and accept new ideas proposed by those in the group itself. When two fans of the same football club discuss something different from sports topics, they presumably do it with a willingness to listen which is different from their attitude when discussing something with a fan of another team. The sense of belonging creates strong bonds, sometimes able to eradicate entrenched opinions.

A dramatic example is the famous one of the *Stanford prison experiment*. For a couple of weeks, without any contact with the outside world, ordinary people without a criminal record impersonated the roles of prison guards and inmates in a simulated prison. The identification with others and the sense of belonging to opposing groups (guards and inmates) was so intense that the experiment had to be interrupted because of the physical and psychological violence of the subjects (Zimbardo 1972).

Although the effects are much less intense, it has been demonstrated that when a computer is given physical superstructures (appearance) and software (communication) which in some way identifies it as "belonging to the same group" as the user, the latter is more willing to interact efficiently with it (Nass, Fogg, Moon 1996).

The sense of belonging to the same group is not true only of the computer, but can be extended to other machines and graphic interfaces. When I go to Croatia and need to draw money in the local currency, I always get a sense of protection and warmth from the fact that the Automated Teller Machine addressed me in Italian. It is not just a question of convenience; English would be perfectly good enough to allow me to draw the money. I think it is rather the fact that it gives me a sense of belonging to my country. Interface with the ATM tells me "You are Italian".

The capacity to converse by imitating the constructs typical of speech is another important element which makes a digital technology a social actor. Most of today's satellite navigators give driving directions in male or female voices which are polite or cheerful, authoritative or accommodating, according to the driver's preferences. Efforts that have been made and which are still being made to 'humanize' synthetic sounds, removing their metallic tone and stiff, unnatural inflections, are not simply for functional reasons. At least, not only. A warm, friendly voice has the power to bring man and machine closer together. The manufacturers of electronic equipment equipped with vocal interface plan their products so that their tone of voice, combined with paralinguistic features (slang, informal expressions, accents) convey, as the case may be, security, deep regret, deference and other moods which are virtually appropriate to the situation. Imagine the following scenario. It is evening and you are worn out after a day's hard work; you long only to close your eyes and sleep, but you still have to do the week's washing. Unfortunately the washing-machine that you have filled with your children's dirty underwear, underwear that will be needed the next day, is blocked by malfunctioning of the water pump. The message you receive is: "The washing-machine has broken down". What would you do? When this happened to me, I kicked it. Now think of the same situation, but with a different ending. Imagine that the washing-machine talks to you in a warm female voice saying how sorry it is: "I am really very sorry. I know full well that this is a serious inconvenience, but there is really nothing I can do about it. There is a malfunctioning that, no matter how much I would like to, I cannot repair." Would your reaction be the same? I doubt it. The tone of voice, its inflections and authoritarian tone are all communicative artifacts to induce irrational behavior.

Despite the fact that it is common knowledge that the quality of verbal communication has significant influence on the quality of inter-action between man and machine, it is not always easy to define beforehand what synthetic sounds need to be used to provoke a specific reaction or produce a predetermined sensation. Consider tone of voice, for example. Is a machine (for example, the washing-machine) more effective in terms of 'acceptability' if it has a voice whose tone is high, innocent and childlike, or a voice with a deeper tone? In an attempt to respond to such questions, some researchers of the University of Twente (The Netherlands) built two "receptionist robots" with different tones of voice and personalities: Olivia, extrovert, lively, with a sense of humour and a high tone of voice, and Cynthia, introvert, calm, more serious and with a decidedly lower tone of voice. The robots were made to interact with a number of subjects. Their tasks were straightforward: make telephone calls, organise appointments, give information, etc. Without going into detail, it emerged that tone of voice greatly influences the judgment of users who give importance to the quality of a service (Niculescu, van Dijk *et al.* 2013).

3. From Expression to Conceptualization: Machines as Social Agents

The saying "never judge a book by its cover" became popular to defend humanity from a significant psychological phenomenon: in the mind of man, at the unconscious level, *a book is judged by its cover*, and nothing could be truer. In their pragmatic spirit, banks to continue to insist on their jacket and tie, knowing that this will transmit a message of relia-bility to their clients. When a shabbily-dressed stranger rings our doorbell, we are suspicious. Judging from appearances is a quick mental calculation which generates immediate, ready-made judgments. At the level of social interaction, the mechanism has its advantages, because here the speed of judgment is more important than its quality. From this point of view, machines and men have several things in common. Badly packaged machines, in inadequate containers and colours inappropriate to context in which they are used, falsify the perception that the user has of their real technical characteristics.

At times, a title or a "qualifying attribute" is enough for a machine to be judged as having better quality. This is the case above all with digital technologies, for those applications that carry out a function which is usually taken care of by a specialist. The app which anyone can download to check the functioning of the batteries of their smartphone is called a *Battery Doctor*. Clearly it does not 'cure' the batteries in any sense. And yet, just because it is honoured by the title 'doctor', it is put on a level that an equivalent app that might be called *Battery Check* could never aspire to. Pay attention to information devices and you will realize that many types of software, from antivirus to online ways of losing weight are given the names of reliable professionals: doctors, policemen, professionals. According to the type of software, it may be described as a 'friend', teacher', 'maestro', and so on.

The psychological effects of the ELIZA software (a *chatbot*) were significant in this respect. This is a software able to impersonate a therapist. The software in question was able to ask questions in writing, addressed to patients, by means of a video terminal. The patients replied by using the same terminal. This made it possible to deliver therapy sessions automatically managed by the machine. The software was written in 1966 by Joseph Weizenbaum when artificial intelligence and chatbots were only just beginning. Weizenbaum was fully aware of the fact that his creation could not replace therapy; it was just as short step ahead in the long journey to artificial intelligence (Weizenbaum 1977). However, the experiments which followed showed that, contrary to this, patients tended to overestimate the role of the software and unknowingly attributed to it a trust similar to that they would have given a flesh-and-blood therapist.

A machine does not even have to be able to talk or resemble a living being in some way to create an emotional contact. It is sufficient for the machine to use a recognized social dynamic. There are various ways in which our interlocutor can be influenced during social interactions, both consciously and unconsciously. When a child wants an ice-cream, the first he does is 'buy' his mother with a kiss. And very often this, and similar kinds of behavior, has the desired effect. In psychology this particular social dynamic is called the *reciprocity principle* (Cialdini 2013): when someone does us a favour, gives us an advantage or is simply kind without necessarily having to be, we feel grateful to that person. Consequently, we feel we should exchange the favour. This is especially true when we confide in someone, whether a friend or not. People are reluctant to divulge information about their personal lives, but there is a kind of implicit rule according to which a person who is confided in feels he should do the same in exchange. There are studies which show that the reciprocity principle can be applied to interaction with computers. In one of these (Nass and Moon 2000), two computers were programmed in such a way as to have different social behaviours. The first was offhand and cold, went straight to the point and asked the subjects questions in an impersonal way. The second computer, instead, revealed something about itself before asking any question. For example, it asked: "At times computers crash for reasons which are incomprehensible in the eyes of their users. This usually happens at the worst possible moment and creates great inconvenience and disappointment. What is there that made you feel most guilty in your life?" The results confirmed that the reciprocity principle is valid also in man–computer interaction. The subjects who interacted with the second computer, in fact, were more willing to share personal details and feelings with the computer. They were aware that they were interacting only with a set of electronic circuits devoid of life and feelings, but some mechanism in their minds made them behave as if they were dealing with a machine which had "something human" about it.

It might seem that computers' ability to influence man is limited and, in any case, that it is not manifested with an intensity so elevated that it is a cause for worry. The truth is that the so-called *persuasive technologies* are widely used in digital applications and make a difference. How often have you received a pop-up message like: "Congratulations, your software has been successfully updated!"? Or messages in which the computer was unnecessarily familiar, calling the user by his first name and praising him, showing that it knew something about his life. On a personal note, every now and then I receive a message along the lines of: "Dear Professor Paolo Gallina, from our research it emerges that the results of your research have positively impressed the scientific community interested in robotics. We would be happy to publish one of your papers in our journal . . . ". These are obviously messages which are automatically pre-packaged for commercial purposes, sent to tens of thousands of professionals most of whom, myself included, make no impression at all on the scientific community. Just the same, messages of this kind generates a feeling of acceptance in the mind which is totally different from that aroused by a cold, impersonal message such as "If you wish, you can publish your research in our journal". It is not true that these forms of technological conditioning appeal only to the minds of unwary users who fall easily for the 'games' of technology. All of us, some more, some less – and the results of experiments confirm this – are vulnerable to the insistence of the techniques of "digital persuasion". We believe ourselves to be more irrational than in fact we are, while instead the inadequacy of irrationality is widely used for profit. Actually the fact that companies in the information industry constantly invest in these areas of research (areas which, for obvious reasons, are never publicized or made public knowledge) is proof that even a simple computer is able to condition the mind and generate *synthetic emotions*.

4. The Imperfect Beauty of Robots

When we pass to anthropomorphic robots, the emotional bond and the production of synthetic emotions is intensified. A personal experience will serve to introduce this part of my essay.

I was in Athens, attending a workshop on robotics and artificial intelligence at the DEMOKRITOS National Center for Research. A professor was about to speak about vision systems in the library hall, and I was early. So I browsed around the next floor where the laboratories were set up. The rooms were empty of people. In a corner of the second laboratory stood a little robot called NOA, a product of the Aldebaran Robotics company. I walked up to it, knelt down, and when the robot perceived my presence by means of its sensors, it was activated, raised its arm and asked: "Would you like to play with me?" I started. On the floor on its right, there were some tennis balls. It probably wanted me to give it one of them. Clearly the robot had been programmed to react in this way. Whether I played or not, it would not have been offended, given that it had not been given any sensibility to arouse offence. And yet at that moment, when I did nothing and stood up, I felt a little uneasy. As if I had disappointed a child. And my feeling of discomfort increased slightly as I went out, when the robot asked: "Eh, you really don't want to play with me?".

If, as we have seen previously, the voice, utterances, expressions, social behavior and roles are characteristics able to create an emotional channel between the user and machines, then giving a machine a human form increases this process of unconscious 'humanization'. The term 'humanization' in this context does not indicate the acquisition by machines of the ontological properties typical (and always exclusive to) human beings. A machine will always be a deterministic set of mechatronic parts. It is the *mind* of man that interacts with the machine which 'humanizes' it. And this process is unconscious. If this were not so, if one had full awareness, instant after instant, of the mechanical nature of the machine, the process would not occur. That our mind behaves in this might be good or not according to the situations and from the cultural point of view with which the phenomenon is analyzed. Anthropomorphism is òne of the many parameters by which a machine can be characterized. It is related to the resemblance between man and machine in question. As a first approximation, it may be stated that the more a robot (in most cases, a machine with an anthropomorphic appearance is a robot) is anthropomorphized, the more it is perceived as an entity between a man and a machine, at least during periods when its rationality is not activated to warn its senses of the deception.

The dichotomy between rationality and irrational emotions in this context must not be underestimated. The intensity of feelings induced by anthropomorphism is high. Very often, users who interact with machines are aware that rationality and emotion come to opposite conclusions: the statement "this is only a machine" comes up beside "this is a machine with something human about it". The interesting and, in many ways, insidious thing is that these two diametrically opposed conclusions go on living in the minds of most users, alternating with the same frequency with which rationality and feelings occur together in daily life. And any attempt to create anything definite between the two positions is doomed to fail.

If it is true that the more a robot, in appearance and kinematically, resembles a human being, the more the mind tends to give it 'human properties', it is also true that this connection is not linear. There is a phenomenon known as the *uncanny valley* (Seyama and Nagayama 2007) which says that if a robot is *almost* a faithful reproduction of a human being, its appearance is grotesque and sinister. It is the *almost* that makes the difference. This is a psychological phenomenon by which the mind perceives an element of danger (for example, associated with a possible disease) if the imperfection disfigures the robot's face. On second thoughts, the phenomenon need not surprise us. Also patients with facial burns, and therefore have skin which is *almost* perfect, at first cause strong emotions and feelings of embarrassment in those who talk to them.

The *uncanny valley* is not the only negative aspect of an excessive resemblance of robot to man. Professor Brian Duffy of the Media Lab Europe in Dublin gives a detailed explanation of how a robot or an interface which employs the advantages if anthropomorphization might be counterproductive in creating a worthwhile interaction with users. The exterior appearance of a machine, in fact, creates expectations which, if not satisfied by the quality of interaction, results in the user's overall negative evaluation (Duffy 2003).

5. Soft and Hard Synthetic Emotions

Phenomena related to the generation of artificial emotions by machines are varied and difficult to classify with any degree of rigour. Furthermore, they are manifested with greatly variable intensity. For this reason, it is appropriate to make a distinction, even if a rough one, between what may be called *soft* and *hard synthetic emotions*.

A computer's ability to make us want to exchange 'kindnesses' is certainly in the category of generating soft synthetic emotions. Of the two, these emotions are the most often studied and exploited for industrial purposes both because they increase profits and because they are easier to generate. *Hard synthetic emotions*, on the other hand, are love, the protective instinct, sense of paternity and so on. Can one fall in love with a machine? Can one develop a feeling so intense that its destruction brings about a sense of confusion? Is it possible to think of a machine in the same way as we think of our child, or, if not our child, at least our dog? It is difficult to give any definite answer which would cover every aspect and doubt that the question raises. But one thing is certain: there exist machines that are able to elicit intense feelings, emotions that we can call *hard synthetic emotions*. In this case too it is dangerous and useless to advance hasty moral judgments. In my view, all that is generated in the human mind is worthy of respect. It goes without saying that respect does not necessarily mean approval.

I have discussed at length in a previous paper, *The Soul of Machines* (Gallina 2015), the mechanisms that permit hard synthetic emotions to be generated in interaction between man and machine. I shall therefore limit myself in what follows to elaborate on that discussion with other aspects which are not usually brought to the fore in dealing with man/robot or man/machine interaction.

6. History, Uniqueness and Unpredictability

In 1891, a worker at the Shelby Electric Company carefully picked up one of the tens of thousands of electric bulbs that the company produced every day and slipped it into a box. On the same day, the owner of the firm, Dennis Bernal, decided to donate the bulb in question to the fire station of Livermore, California (http://www.centennial-

bulb.org/). *It was a bulb like any other, except for the fact that, one hundred years later, it continue to give out a feeble light while hanging from an electric wire. When, a few years ago, it was temporarily switched off to allow maintenance to be carried out on the electric plant, the technicians were left with bated breath. It was as if the bulb had been subjected to delicate surgery. Today, those who have grown fond of it expect the carbon bulb, given its age, to stop giving out that old light, recalling a death rattle. And they await this event with a kind of sad resignation. Why all this attention and apprehension? Why has the bulb managed to generate hard synthetic emotions? There is nothing wrong in talking about hard emotions in this case. The bulb, and only that bulb, has no persuasive function which could reproduce human communication for commercial gain; that bulb, and only that bulb, possesses the unique power to generate affection. It might be very slight, but it is genuine, unreasoning affection.*

Why? First of all, its resistance over the years is a metaphor of life, its feeble flicker is a metaphor

for old age and the day it switches off will be a metaphor for death. And even this would be enough to overcome the difficulties of anthropofiltre. But this parallel of stages of human life and the cycle of the life of the product will not explain the intensity of the phenomenon. After all, every light bulb is made, works for a while and, sooner or later, wears out. What makes the difference in this case is time. Man gives great importance to the fact of "having lived and experienced". History makes objects more precious and sometimes makes them worthy of occupying prestigious pedestals in museums.

In debates on artificial intelligence, the question is asked if, in future, we will believe that robots equipped with an intelligence comparable or superior to our own are alive.

The discriminating factor, what separates artificial life from non-artificial life is the power of evaluation. I personally think that this is a limited way of looking at things and, for this reason, misleading. To consider or not to consider something as having life, or rather, to perceive that something inanimate is living, involves the cognitive dimension of the mind only in part. It is mainly the emotions which govern our convictions regarding the attribution of life. And the emotions are generated by attributes of the machine that do not always have something to do with intelligence. This question of "having experienced" is one of these. But what is meant by "having experienced"? And in what way can a robot or an artificial intelligence said to live?

Suppose there is Superbrain, an electric brain similar to that of a living being. Superbrain is able to respond to any of our questions, any query, and has no problem having a conversation. The problem is that today's Superbrain is identical to yesterday's Superbrain and that of the day before. Men and animals never remain identical to themselves. They change over time. *Change* is the clearest of all evidence that we are alive. And this evidence is *irreversible*: there is no turning back. Experience and time leave an indelible impression on us. If a machine, no matter how intelligent, is unable to change and is incapable of irreversibility, it cannot hope to induce feelings similar to those one feels for a living being.

For better or worse, robots or digital agents which implement and fully simulate life in these terms have not yet been devised. Every robot can be reset whenever it needs to be. It can therefore be reborn innumerable times and this property means that it is an object that can be remade in exactly the same form, devoid of the magic and fascination of the natural.

7. Mediator Machines in Interpersonal Relationships

Hard synthetic emotions do not arise exclusively from the interaction between a single man and a machine. They can be generated also in those situations in which a machine *mediates* communication between one user and another, or between one user and many others.

In order to understand these forms of synthetic emotions, we have to start from a statement which is as banal as it is necessary: put plainly and simply, many people believe that humanity, in its biological and social nature, is highly unsatisfactory. The rest maintain, on the contrary, that the world is rich in opportunities to achieving that happiness that the others believe unattainable. Usually the latter criticize the former for expressing judgments that are too categorical and negative regarding humanity as a whole. Furthermore, they interpret the awareness of dissatisfaction of a living being as an anomaly, an exception that must be fought against and cared about, and not as the result of a reflection on man's biological nature. Despite the fact that I personally support the ideas that society and every single individual should make an attempt to make life tolerable, I am convinced that the origin of the dynamism of living beings is to be found in dissatisfaction. We live in a very imperfect world. And even if we should reach perfection in terms of justice, health, politics and the redistribution of resources, we shall continue to feel a sense of incompleteness. It is in the nature of our being dynamic beings to be dissatisfied. To feel totally fulfilled would mean not having any reason to act and, therefore, would lead to aphasia.

It is the feeling for this kind of environment that the MMORPG (*Massively Multiplayer Online Role-Playing Game*) and the MUVE (*Multi-User Virtual Environments*) are becoming more and more popular. The first are videogames or role-plays played online, in which thousands of players can interact by playing a specific role (character) whose actions are reflected in the dynamic of the game which is characterized by a setting. In the case of *Warcraft*, for example, the players 'live' in a fantasy world inhabited by ogres, knights and other legendary characters.

When studying these social phenomena, it is important to start from the premise that in modern society, so intensely innervated by technology, virtual worlds are a alternative to real life or at least attempts at alternatives to real life. It has in fact been amply demonstrated that users choose to impersonate roles whose characteristics reflect their ideal desired way of life which is denied by the reality in which they live (Bessiére, Seay, Kiesler 2007).

These virtual settings allow us to overcome the limits of the real which imposes on us bodies from the moment of birth whose attraction is not often that which the owner wishes for (such dissatisfaction is also true of a not-insignificant percentage of those who spend time in virtual worlds such as *Second Life*). Taking on the appearance of an avatar allows us to approach virtual couples which often develop in a relation in the real world.

I imagine that, for every couple who fall in love in the virtual world and continues to keep up the relationship in the real world, there is another who, having to face up to harsh reality, fall out without each other and see no similarity to the virtual world. This does not mean that the phenomenon is numerically significant and draws life from the ability of machines to generate synthetic feelings in an activity of mediation. In this case too, it is the machine which generates synthetic emotions, a machine which cheats the mind. Cheating in this context is not to be interpreted in its negative sense. Cheating is usually an expression of the fact that some emotions would never occur without the machine's mediation, entrusting themselves to nature. The MUVE are able to amplify a living being's capacity to appear better than in fact he is. A centralized server collects information inserted in real time and transforms it into virtual scenarios, behaviours and actions which are made available to the remote user. The words typed onto the keyboard become the voice of an avatar. And this continual scene, unreal but fascinating, plants powerful suggestions into the mind of the user.

To understand the mechanisms of falling in love in virtual worlds, we should start from falling in love in the real world. Firstly, we have to accept a truth: however wrong it might be, however open to criticism, cynical, insensitive, unjust it might be and not matter our sense of civilization tends to think the opposite, the number of men who are attracted by "the beauty that a woman has inside" are few. In order to reach a man's heart, the woman must first overcome the attraction filter. This filter carries out a strict selection and works for a short time. When the woman has passed the test" of the attraction filter, the real relationship of the couple begins and they begin to get to know each other. It is only then that the man discovers and appreciates (or not) interior beauty. Therefore, to finally conquer the man's heart, the woman has to pass through a second filter, the filter we can call the *introspective filter*. It goes without saying that the man has to pass through the same filters in the same order in order to reach the woman's heart.

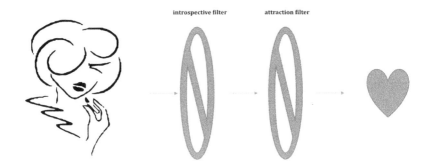

These filters are active also in virtual world where men and women impersonate unreal avatars. The process is similar, but with one basic difference: the filters' position is inverted.

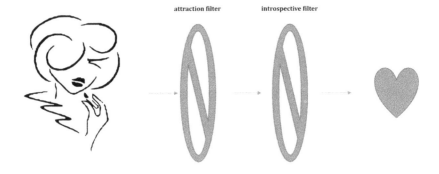

The avatars of *Second Life* are all more or less beautiful and fascinating. Few of them, above all those looking for their soulmate, are interested in taking the part of an ugly, awkward and overweight character. The effect of this levelling to absolute standards of beauty is that the user, in order to reach the heart of another user, finds it easy to overcome the attraction filter (which operates in the virtual environment). In effect, it is as if this filter were not active. Their meeting is therefore more due to chance than to choice. Having met, the users begin to get to know each other and this knowledge develops on the cognitive level. As they exchange textual and spoken messages which are the expression of true interiority, the introspective filter begins to reject and approve. When, but only later, the two users meet in flesh and blood, the attraction filter – now in the real world – has the last word in approving the relationship or otherwise. This explains why some couples who meet in the virtual world choose to continue their relationship in the real world. Furthermore, it should be noted that overcoming the test of the introspective filter guarantees a stability which is much longer-lasting than that obtained by the attraction filter. In other words, we tire of external beauty long before interior beauty.

The two filters have no way of communicating between them: inversion of these filters does not produce the same result. It need not be true that two people united in love sparked off in the virtual world have the same chances in the real one and vice versa.

Bibliography

Barnes, S., Pressey, A. 2014: Caught in the Web? Addictive Behavior in Cyberspace and the Role of Goal-orientation. *Technological Forecasting and Social Change* 86, 93–109.

Bessiére, K., Seay, A., Kiesler, S. 2007: The Ideal Self: Identity Exploration in World of Warcraft. *Cyberpsychology and Behavior* 10 (4), 530–535.

Cialdini, R. B. 2006: *Influence. The Psychology of Persuasion,* (revisited edition). HarperCollins: New York.

Duffy, B. R. 2003: Anthropomorphism and the Social Robot. *Robotics and Autonomous Systems.* 42 (4), 177–190.

Fogg, B. J. 2002: *Persuasive Technology: Using Computers to Change What We Think and Do.* Burlington (MA): Morgan Kaufmann.

Fogg, B. J., and Nass, C. 1997: Silicon Sycophants: The Effects of Computers That Flatter. *International Journal of Human Computer Studies* 46 (5), 551–561.

Gallina, P. 2015: *L'anima delle macchine. Tecnodestino, dipendenza tecnologica e uomo virtuale.* Bari: Dedalo.

Herodotou, C., Kambouri, M., Winters, N. 2014: Dispelling the Myth of the Socio-emotionally Dissatisfied Gamer. *Computers in Human Behavior* 32, 23–31.

Kardefelt-Winther, D. 2014: The Moderating Role of Psychosocial Well-being on the Relationship Between Escapism and Excessive Online Gaming. *Computers in Human Behavior* 38, 68–74.

Leménager, T., Dieter, J., Hill, H., *et al.* 2014: Neurobiological Correlates of Physical Self-concept and Self-identification With Avatars in Addicted Players of Massively Multiplayer Online Role-Playing Games (MMORPGs). *Addictive Behaviors* 39 (12), 1789–1797.

Nass, C., Fogg, B. J., Moon, Y. 1996: Can Computers be Teammates? *International Journal of Human-Computer Studies* 45, 669–678.

Nass, C., and Moon, Y. 2000: Machines and Mindlessness: Social Responses to Computers. *Journal of Social Issues* 56 (1), 81–103.

Niculescu, A., van Dijk B. *et al.* 2013: Making Social Robots More Attractive: The Effect of Voice Pitch, Humor and Empathy. *International Journal of Social Robotics* 5 (2), 171–191.

Seyama, J. and Nagayama, R. S. 2007: The Uncanny Valley: Effect of Realism on the Impression of Artificial Human Faces. *Presence* 16 (4), 337–351.

Sullins, J. 2012: Robots, Love, and Sex: The Ethics of Building a Love Machine. *IEEE Transactions on Affective Computing* 3 (4), 398–409.

Weizenbaum, J. 1977: *Computer Power and Human Reason: From Judgment To Calculation.* San Francisco: Freeman.

The Editors and Contributors

The Editors

MAURO MALDONATO is an italian psychiatrist, professor at University of Basilicata. He has been a visiting professor at Duke University, at Universidade de São Paulo (USP) and Pontifícia Universidade Católica (PUC) of São Paulo. He is an author and curator of volumes and scientific articles published in numerous languages. He is also the scientific director of International Research Week.

PAOLO AUGUSTO MASULLO, Ph.D., is an italian philosopher, professor and director of the Department of Human Sciences at University of Basilicata. He has studied Max Scheler and the Phenomenological Movement, Viktor von Weizsäcker and his philosophy of medicine, and the anthropological category of posthuman. He is author of numerous essays and articles and has translated some important works of Viktor von Weizsäcker.

The Contributors

RADWA KHALIL is a Ph.D. candidate in Neuroscience at the Rutgers University. Her research interests are focused on neurobiological/psychological processes and mental and neuro-economic theories underlying specific human behaviours.

SILVIA DELL'ORCO Ph.D., is an italian psychologist. Her research is conducted in the field of the psychology of reasoning and decision making, cognitive neuroscience and clinical psychology. She is author and co-author of many articles in scientific journals.

ROBERTA BARNI is an Italian professor of literature and literary translation at the Faculty of Philosophy, Languages and Human Sciences of the University of São Paulo (USP), Brazil. Her main interests are on multidisciplinary approaches to literature and other art expressions, and on neurosciences and the aesthetic experience of narrative. She is the author of many essays and scientific articles published in Brazil and Italy.

She has translated over 50 books of Italian literature, mainly into Portuguese.

RAFFAELE SPERANDEO Ph.D., is an italian Psychiatrist, Psychotherapist, Professor and Director of SiPGI (School of Gestalt Psychotherapy Integrated). He is author and co-author of many articles in scientific journals

LUDOVICA TREMANTE is an italian psychologist and psychoterapist in training. She is also a teacher of Human Sciences at high school.

SANTO DI NUOVO, Ph.D. and Psy.D., is an Italian psychologist, professor and director of the Department of Education at University of Catania, and President of the Academy of Fine Arts of Catania. He has cooperated in an international research group on the applications of neurosciences with the Center for Robotics and Neural System of the University of Plymouth (UK). He is author or co-author of many articles and books on methodological and applicative issues in different field of psychology and rehabilitation.

DANIELA CONTI graduated with BSc and MSc in Psychology and BSc in Psychiatric Rehabilitation and Social Education and received the Ph.D. in Neuroscience at University of Catania, Italy. From 2013 to 2015 she was visiting at Plymouth University (UK), Centre for Robotics and Neural Systems. Currently she is Marie Curie Research Fellow at Sheffield Hallam University (UK). Her main research interests are focused on application of cognitive robotics to diagnosis of intellectual disability and psychiatric rehabilitation.

ALESSANDRO DI NUOVO received the MSc and Ph.D. degrees in computer engineering from the University of Catania, Italy, in 2005 and 2009, respectively. He is currently Senior Lecturer at Sheffield Hallam University (UK) and engaged in teaching activities at the University of Enna (Italy). His research specializes in computational intelligence and its application to cognitive robotics, human–robot interaction, computer-aided assessment of intellectual disabilities, and embedded computer systems. He is author of over 70 scientific articles and he was involved in many European research projects and networks.

PAOLO VALERIO is a Clinical Psychologist, Psychodynamic Psychotherapist. Full professor of Clinical Psychology at the Naples University Federico II Medical School. Author and co-author of books and of scientific articles published in Italian and international journals. His area of research is about gender identity, gender dysphorias, sexual orientations, homo/transphobia, intersexualities, gender based violence. He is President of the "National Observatory on Gender Identity" (ONIG) and of the Foundation "Gender Identity and Culture"

ROBERTO VITELLI is Assistant Professor in Clinical Psychology at the Federico II University of Naples. He is co-founder of the Gender Dysphoria Psychological Service, run since 1997 by the Federico II University Hospital. He is a Fellow of the Italian Psychological Association – Clinical and Dynamic Section and of the UK Sartre Society. He is a member and co-founder of the School for Psychotherapy and Clinical Phenomenology – Florence (Italy). He is editor of several books and author of many scientific articles.

DARIO GIUGLIANO Ph.D., is an Italian philosopher. He lives in Naples, where he works as professor of aesthetics at the Academy of Fine Arts. His most recent book, *Il discorso sospeso: sul corpo dell'arte* (2003), examines visual arts, philosophy and corporality. He is editor of the journal "estetica: studi e ricerche" and member of the Advisory Board of the journal "Third Text" and foreign member of the Accademia di Scienze Morali e Politiche of the Società Nazionale di Scienze Lettere e Arti in Napoli. He has recently published essays on Gilles Deleuze and Martin Heidegger in "Rue Descartes" and "Etica & Politica/Ethics & Politics" respectively, and on Pier Paolo Pasolini in "Third Text".

AGOSTINO CERA is Adjunct Professor of Theoretical Philosophy at the University of Basilicata. He works on and has published in Continental philosophy between XIX and XX century (especially on Karl Löwith), philosophical anthropology and philosophy of technology.

ANNA DONISE is University Professor of Moral Philosophy (University of Naples – Federico II). Her research focuses on neokantianism (Rickert) and phenomenology (Husserl, Scheler, Jaspers). She is presently working on the role of the imagination and of the emotive sphere in determining actions. She is the author of many volumes and essays, and has translated into Italian works of Edmund Husserl and Karl Jaspers.

ROSSELLA CORDA Ph.D. in Philosophy (University of Bari), currently Ph.D. student in "History and literature" at the University of Basilicata. She is author of several papers about the philosophy of Gilles Deleuze and F. Guattari.

PAOLO GALLINA is currently associate professor of Applied Mechanics at the Department of Civil Engineering and Architecture, University of Trieste, Trieste (Italy). He was visiting professor at the Ohio University in 2000/1. In 2002 he implemented a hands-on Mechatornic Laboratory for students in Engineering. In 2003 he implemented a Robotics Laboratory where he carries out his main research in robotics. In 2004 he was visiting professor at the Colorado University, at the "Center for Advanced Manufacturing and Packaging of Microwave, Optical and Digital Electronics", in order to collaborate on mechatronics and micromechanics fields. He was head of the Council for Students in Mechanical Engineering Degree from 2004 to 2008. Head of the master's program: "Safety and hygiene in the working environment" from 2006 to 2008. His interests are in vibrations, human–machine interfaces, robotics, especially applied to rehabilitation.

Subject Index